Spiral CT
of the Body

Spiral CT of the Body

A Teaching File

R. BROOKE JEFFREY, JR.

Professor of Radiology
Chief of Abdominal Imaging
Stanford University Medical Center

ELLIOT K. FISHMAN

Professor of Radiology and Oncology
Johns Hopkins School of Medicine

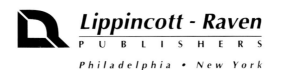

Lippincott - Raven
PUBLISHERS

Philadelphia • New York

Acquisitions Editor: Jim Ryan
Development Editor: Karen Frame
Manufacturing Manager: Dennis Teston
Production Manager: Larry Bernstein
Production Editor: Dee Josephson
Cover Designer: Ede Dreikers
Indexer: Susan Thomas
Compositor: Maryland Composition
Printer: Courier-Westford

Printed in the United States of America

9 8 7 6 5 4 3 2 1

Library of Congress Cataloging-in-Publication Data
Spiral CT of the body: a teaching file / edited by R. Brooke Jeffrey and Elliott
  Fishman.
        p.   cm.
    Includes bibliographical references and index.
    ISBN 0-397-51668-1 (case)
    1. Spiral computed tomography. I. Jeffrey, R. Brooke
II. Fishman, Elliot K.
    [DNLM: 1. Tomography, R-Ray Computed—methods.   WN 206 S759 1996]
RC78.7.T6S647   1996
616.07′52-dc20
DNLM/DLC
for Library of Congress

To
Stefanie, Catherine, Luke, and Elizabeth
R. Brooke Jeffrey, Jr.

To
Whitney, Torrey, and Lori
Elliot K. Fishman

Contents

PREFACE ix

ACKNOWLEDGMENTS x

Section 1
The Cardiovascular System 1

Section 2
The Chest 59

Section 3
The Gall Bladder and Bile Ducts 121

Section 4
The Gastrointestinal Tract 127

Section 5
The Genitourinary Tract 171

Section 6
The Kidneys and Adrenal Glands 185

Section 7
The Liver 211

Section 8
The Musculoskeletal System 259

Section 9
The Pancreas 271

Section 10
The Retroperitoneum 305

Section 11
The Spleen 313

INDEX 323

The development of spiral (helical) CT represents a major technical advance in body imaging. By combining a continuous gantry rotation with a continuous table feed, spiral scanning eliminates inter-scan delay. This enables spiral CT scan acquisitions to be up to nine times faster than conventional or dynamic CT. For the first time, breathheld imaging of major regions of the body such as the chest and abdomen are now routine. The advantage of breathheld imaging is that CT data sets can be obtained free of motion and respiratory artifacts that can be edited using a variety of sophisticated techniques. This greatly facilitates accurate display of vascular anatomy with three-dimensional CT angiography. In addition, the speed of spiral CT allows scan acquisition during peak contrast enhancement of the target organ, thus improving evaluation of a variety of visceral disorders.

The purpose of this book is to highlight the imaging advantages of spiral CT emphasizing its unique technical and clinical features. It is not, therefore, intended as a comprehensive review of pathology of the chest and abdomen. Specific examples have been selected to showcase the clinical utility of spiral CT emphasizing such new techniques as biphasic scanning (arterial- and venous-phase imaging), three-dimensional CT angiography, multiplanar reconstructions and optimization of scan acquisition during the contrast bolus. It is our hope that this case presentation format will provide a greater understanding of the technical aspects of CT that can be used in clinical practice.

Acknowledgment

I am very grateful to my secretary Kevin Murphy for his outstanding editorial assistance in the preparation of this manuscript. In addition I would like to thank the Residents, Fellows, and CT technologists at Stanford for their enthusiasm, hard work, and diligence in helping me to collect cases for this project.

SECTION 1

The Cardiovascular System

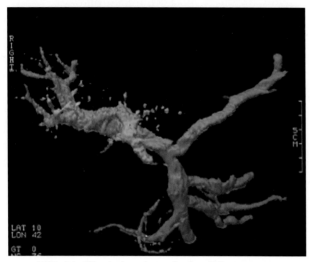

FIG. 1A. Shaded-surface display CT venogram

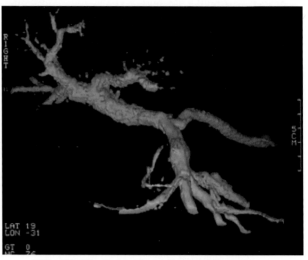

FIG. 1B. Shaded-surface display CT venogram

History

Pancreatic carcinoma. Rule out venous occlusion.

Findings

Figures 1A and B are venous-phase shaded-surface display images obtained from a spiral CT venogram of the upper abdomen. Note the patency of the superior mesenteric splenic and portal veins. Multiple jejunal branches are well visualized on the shaded surface displays.

Diagnosis

Normal portal venous system demonstrated by CT venography.

Discussion

Excellent images of the portal venous system may be obtained with spiral CT venography. Acquisition is delayed for approximately 45 seconds following the intravenous injection of contrast medium, in order to maximize enhancement during the peak phase of venous opacification. Either shaded surface displays or maximum intensity projections (MIP) are useful for displaying the venous anatomy. The coronal display simulates the venous phase of a celiac arteriogram and is often easily interpreted by pancreatic surgeons.

References

Balm R, Eikelboom BC, van Leeuwen MS, Noordzij J. Spiral CT-angiography of the aorta. *Eur J Vasc Surg* 1994; 8:544–551.

Semba CP, Rubin GD, Dake MD. Three-dimensional spiral CT angiography of the abdomen. *Semin Ultrasound CT MR* 1994; 15:133–138.

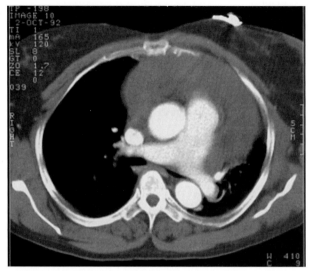

FIG. 2A. Contrast-enhanced CT

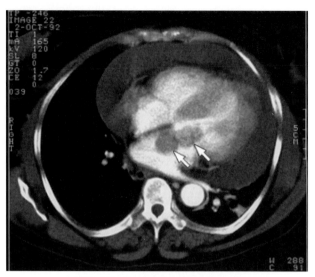

FIG. 2B. Contrast-enhanced CT

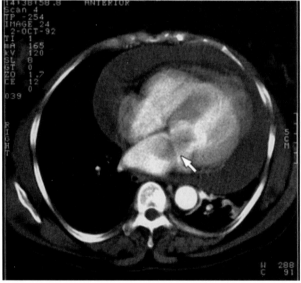

FIG. 2C. Contrast-enhanced CT

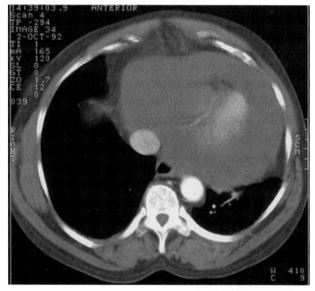

FIG. 2D. Contrast-enhanced CT

History

A 50-year-old female with a history of increased shortness of breath and dyspnea. A routine chest x-ray demonstrated mediastinal widening. A spiral CT was requested for further evaluation.

Findings

A spiral CT scan demonstrates a large filling defect in the left atrium (arrows) near the wall of the arterial septum. The mass is inhomogeneous and is hypodense relative to enhanced blood in the cardiac chambers. There is also a pericardial effusion, as well as a small left pneumothorax.

Diagnosis

Atrial myxoma.

Discussion

The study of choice for the evaluation of a suspected cardiac mass is magnetic resonance imaging (MRI). However, cardiac tumors may be unsuspected findings, as in the current case. In these cases, spiral CT with rapid data acquisition during the phase of cardiac chamber enhancement would probably detect and define the presence of intracardiac masses. This is especially true when data acquisition times of 0.5 to 0.75 seconds per scan are used.

The most common cardiac tumor is a metastasis, often secondary to a lung or breast tumor, lymphoma, leukemia, or melanoma. Primary cardiac tumors are rare, and the majority are benign. In fact, only about 23% of primary cardiac tumors are malignant. Myxomas account for about 25% of the benign tumors, with most tumors arising in the left atrium.

Tsuchiya reviewed 13 cases of atrial myxoma and found them to range in size from about 4 to 8 cm in maximum dimension. The CT appearance was typically inhomogeneous, and the tumors were hypodense relative to the enhanced cardiac chambers. Calcification may be present. The tumor typically arises in or near the fossa ovale of the atrial septum. Most of these tumors are pedunculated.

The CT appearance and location of the tumor mass can usually allow its differentiation from intracardiac thrombus. Thrombus tends to occur in the posterior and lateral wall of the left atrium. Differentiation from cardiac sarcomas or metastasis may, however, be more difficult.

In the case presented, the location of the mass, its enhancement pattern, and its inhomogeneity are most consistent with the key diagnosis of atrial myxoma.

References

McAllister HA Jr, Fenoglio JJ Jr. Tumors of the cardiovascular system. In *Atlas of tumor pathology*. Second series, Fasc. 15. Washington DC: AFIP 1978:1–3.

Steiner MR, Flicker S, Eldredge WJ, et al. Clinical experience with rapid acquisition cardiovascular CT imaging (cine CT) in the adult patient. *RadioGraphics* 1989; 9:283–305.

Tsuchiya F, Kohno A, Saitoh R, Shigeta A. CT findings of atrial myxoma. *Radiology* 1984; 153:139–143.

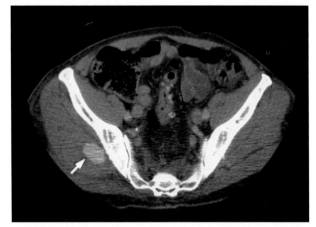

FIG. 3A. Contrast-enhanced CT

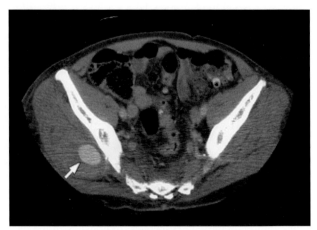

FIG. 3B. Contrast-enhanced CT

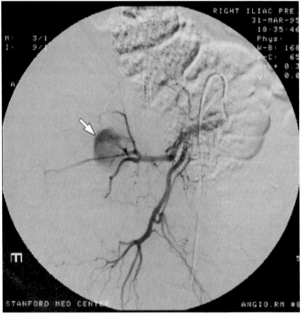

FIG. 3C. Angiogram[3:103/153|]

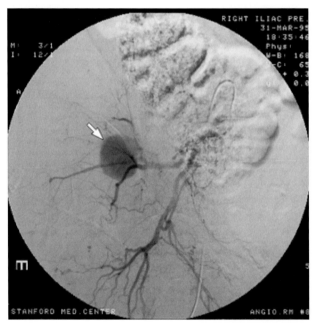

FIG. 3D. Angiogram[3:110/151|]

History

Right buttock pain and hematoma following right iliac bone-marrow harvesting for bone-marrow transplantation.

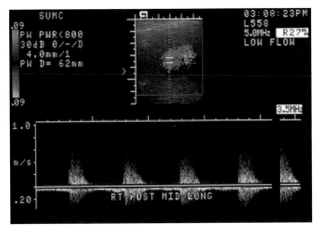

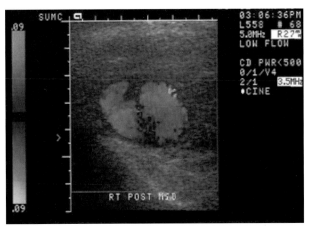

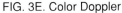

FIG. 3E. Color Doppler   FIG. 3F. Color Doppler

Findings

Figures 3A and 3B are contrast-enhanced spiral CT scans of the pelvis demonstrating an enhancing pseudoaneurysm in the right gluteal area (arrow). This is confirmed angiographically in Figure 3C and D. The color Doppler images also demonstrate the pseudoaneurysm.

Diagnosis

Right gluteal pseudoaneurysm following bone-marrow biopsy.

Discussion

This patient presented with a painful right buttock hematoma following bone-marrow harvesting. A pseudoaneurysm was not clinically suspected. The excellent vascular opacification with spiral CT established the diagnosis of a pseudoaneurysm in the right gluteal region. This was successfully embolized on the same day it was detected.

References

Calligaro KD, Savarese RP, Goldberg D, Doerr KJ, Dougherty MJ, DeLaurentis DA. Deep femoral artery pseudoaneurysm caused by acute trunk and hip torsion. *Cardiovasc Surg* 1993; 1:392–394.

Fujiwara T, Tanohata K, Nagase M. Pseudoaneurysm caused by acupuncture: a rare complication (Letter). *AJR* 1994; 162:731.

Kurihashi A, Tamai K, Saotome K. Peroneal arteriovenous fistula and pseudoaneurysm formation after blunt trauma. A case report. *Clin Orthopaed Rel Res* 1994; 304:Jul:218–221.

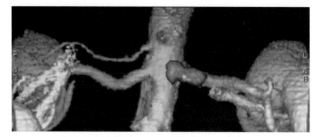

FIG. 4A. 3D CT

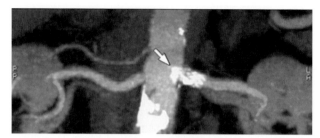

FIG. 4B. MIP

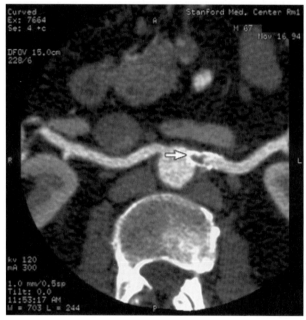

FIG. 4C. Reformatted CT

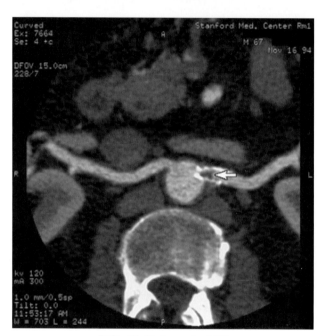

FIG. 4D. Reformatted CT

History

Patient who had placement of an intrarenal stent for renovascular hypertension. The patient now has elevated blood pressure. Rule out restenosis.

Findings

Figure 4A is a shaded-surface display in a coronal plane of the renal arteries. Note that there are two renal arteries on the right and a single renal artery on the left. The area of increased density overlying the proximal left renal artery is due to a metal artifact from the renal-artery stent. Figure 4B is a maximum-intensity projection (MIP) obtained of the renal arteries, demonstrating calcification in the aorta and a metallic stent in the proximal left renal artery (arrow). Notice that the stent protrudes into the aorta. Figure 4C and D are curved planar reformations through the plane of the stent, demonstrating narrowing of the stent at the aortic orifice and intraluminal low-density thrombus (arrow) within the stent.

Diagnosis

Thrombus identified within a renal-artery stent on curved planar reformation.

Discussion

Evaluation of the renal arteries is one of the main clinical applications of three-dimensional CT angiography. However, in order to adequately display the renal arteries, it is often necessary to perform multiple types of editing and imaging reformation. In addition to shaded-surface displays and MIPs, it is often extremely valuable to perform curved planar reformations. Curved planar reformations are generally 1-pixel thick scans that are prescribed from axial images of the renal arteries. This method of editing has the advantage of demonstrating the internal lumen of metallic endoluminal devices such as stents and stent grafts. In this case, the internal thrombus inside the renal-artery stent could only be displayed by the curved planar reformation. The patient was subsequently treated with balloon angioplasty to reopen the stent, and this proved successful.

References

Balm R, Eikelboom BC, van Leeuwen MS, Noordzij J. Spiral CT-angiography of the aorta. *Eur J Vasc Surg* 1994; 8:544–551.

Semba CP, Rubin GD, Dake MD. Three-dimensional spiral CT angiography of the abdomen. *Semin Ultrasound CT MR* 1994; 15:133–138.

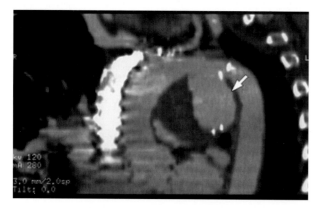

FIG. 5A. Curved reformation

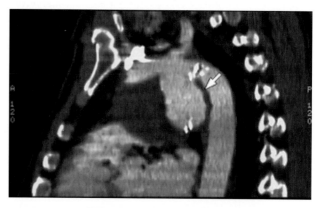

FIG. 5B. Sagittal reformation

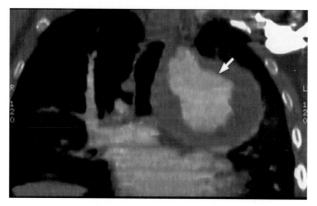

FIG. 5C. Coronal reformation

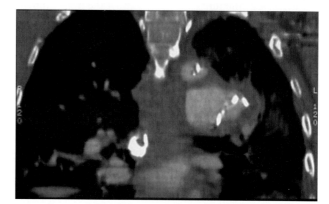

FIG. 5D. Coronal reformation

History

Fever and mediastinal mass.

Findings

Figures 5A–D are sagittal and coronal reformations obtained after a three-dimensional spiral CT angiogram (CTA) of the thoracic aorta. Note on all four images the large saccular aneurysm (arrow) involving the transverse portion of the aortic arch. There is extensive mural thrombus within the aneurysm.

Diagnosis

Mycotic aneurysm of the thoracic aorta.

Discussion

Mycotic aneurysms must always be kept in mind in patients with fever, infective endocarditis, and evidence of an abdominal or thoracic aneurysm. Luetic aortitis most often involves the ascending aorta. Other causes of mycotic aneurysms of the ascending aorta include infection at the suture line following aortic surgery. Aneurysms associated with bacterial infection (in this case due to *Salmonella*) may involve many other segments of the aorta and its branches. Not infrequently, the lower descending and upper lumbar aorta are involved with mycotic aneurysms. The CTA clearly demonstrated the residual lumen and thrombus in this patient, as well as the relationship of the aneurysm to the subclavian and left carotid arteries on the sagittal reformations.

References

McGiffin DC, Galbraith AJ, McCarthy JB, Tesar PJ. Mycotic false aneurysm of the aortic suture line after heart transplantation. *J Heart Lung Transplant* 1994; 13:926–928.

Molina PL, Strobl PW, Burstain JM. Aortoesophageal fistula secondary to mycotic aneurysm of the descending thoracic aorta: CT demonstration. *J Comput Assist Tomogr* 1995 19:309–311.

Sing TM, Young N, O'Rourke IC, Tomlinson P. Leaking mycotic abdominal aortic aneurysm. *Australasian Radiol* 1994; 38:310–312.

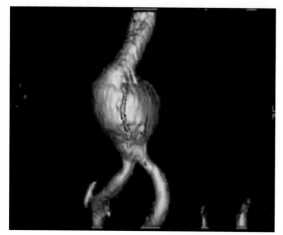

FIG. 6A. 3D CT

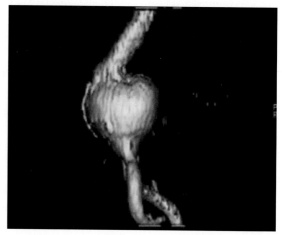

FIG. 6B. 3D CT

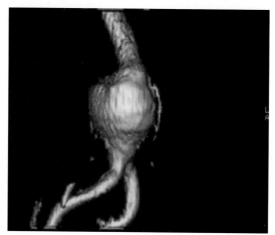

FIG. 6C. 3D CT

History

Preoperative evaluation for abdominal aortic aneurysm.

Findings

Figures 6A–C are shaded-surface displays obtained from a three-dimensional spiral CT angiogram of the aorta. Note the saccular aneurysm of the distal aorta well below the renal arteries. The inferior mesenteric artery is well-visualized in Figure 6B and C, and originates from the aorta anteriorly at the superior margin of the aneurysm. The aneurysm does not extend to the iliac arteries.

Diagnosis

Intrarenal abdominal aortic aneurysm.

Discussion

The preoperative evaluation of an abdominal aortic aneurysm can be done with conventional angiography, magnetic resonance imaging (MRI), or three-dimensional CT angiography (CTA). The primary goals of imaging are to determine the level of the aneurysm and the extent of the involvement of the renal and iliac arteries. MRI is preferred in patients with impaired renal function because it can be performed either without contrast enhancement or with gadolinium, which has no effect on renal function. In patients with normal renal function, CTA is an excellent study to evaluate abdominal aortic aneurysms because of its high degree of spatial resolution.

References

Balm R, Eikelboom BC, van Leeuwen MS, Noordzij J. Spiral CT-angiography of the aorta. *Eur J Vasc Surg* 1994; 8:544–551.

Semba CP, Rubin GD, Dake MD. Three-dimensional spiral CT angiography of the abdomen. *Semin Ultrasound CT MR* 1994; 15:133–138.

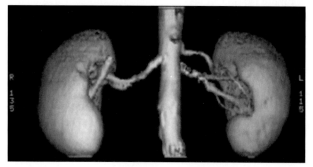

FIG. 7A. 3D CT

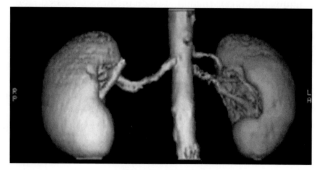

FIG. 7B. 3D CT

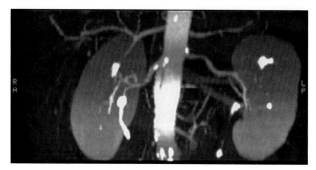

FIG. 7C. MIP

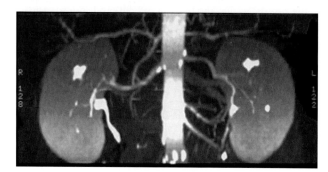

FIG. 7D. MIP

History

Preoperative evaluation for a living, related renal transplant donor.

Findings

Figures 7A and B are shaded-surface displays from a three-dimensional CT angiogram. Note the single renal artery on the right, but two vascular structures in the left renal hilum.

Figure 7C and D are MIP projections from the same data set demonstrating that there is a single left renal artery and that the inferior structure in the left renal hilum is the renal vein.

Diagnosis

Normal bilateral renal arteries in a renal transplant donor.

Discussion

In selective patients, three-dimensional CT angiography plus a digital image of the renal collecting systems may replace the standard workup for living-related donor transplantation, involving abdominal aortography and intravenous pyelography. When transplant surgeons evaluate the kidneys of a living related donor, the left kidney is generally the preferred organ for transplantation because of the longer segment of the left renal vein. However, vascular anomalies, including multiple renal arteries or early branching of renal arteries, preclude transplantation. In this patient the left renal vein was overlying the renal hilum on the shaded-surface display. The MIP projection shows that the vein is clearly of lower attenuation than the artery. A small fleck of calcification can be seen at the origin of the left renal artery as well. Therefore, it is essential to use more than one mode of editing to evaluate the renal arteries, in order to avoid potential misdiagnoses. Also evident on the MIP projection are symmetric nephrograms with early filling of the collecting system. However, a delayed film taken at approximately 10 minutes, using a digital scout radiograph, is optimal for evaluating the renal collecting systems.

References

Alfrey EJ, Rubin GD, Kuo PC, et al. The use of spiral computed tomography in the evaluation of living donors for kidney transplantation. *Transplantation* 1995; 59:643–645.

Mell MW, Alfrey EJ, Rubin GD, Scandling JD, Jeffrey RB Jr, Dafoe DC. Use of spiral computed tomography in the diagnosis of transplant renal stenosis. *Transplantation* 1994; 57:746–779.

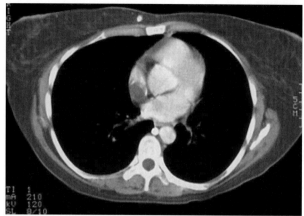

FIG. 8A. Contrast-enhanced CT

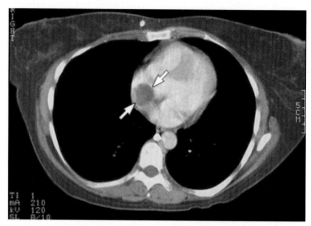

FIG. 8B. Contrast-enhanced CT

History

A 40-year-old female with increasing abdominal girth and a history of cirrhotic liver disease.

Findings

A spiral CT scan demonstrates a filling defect in the right atrium. Scans through the upper abdomen demonstrated cirrhosis of the liver with ascites. A Leveen shunt was also seen.

Diagnosis

Right atrial mass due to organizing thrombus.

Discussion

Although MRI is the study of choice for evaluation of cardiac pathology, CT will often detect unsuspected cardiac disease, as in the present case. With the use of spiral CT during optimal phases of contrast enhancement, it is not surprising that vascular pathology, particularly involving thrombosis, is seen more frequently. The detection of thrombus is related in most cases to the relative enhancement of the surrounding structures and the lack of enhancement of the thrombus. In the present case, enhancement of the cardiac chamber is well seen, and a 2-cm low-density area in the right atrium, consistent with a thrombus, was noted. Although the entire chest was not scanned in this examination, the thrombus was found at surgery to extend into the superior vena cava. The cause of the thrombus was never absolutely determined.

Filling defects in the heart can be due to primary or metastatic tumors. Specifically, filling defects in the right atrium can be due to a tumor such as an atrial myxoma. The possibility of metastatic disease should be a consideration, but it is uncommon. An atrial thrombus may become a source of embolic phenomena. In the present case the patient's clinical symptoms were probably related to the underlying cirrhosis and ascites rather than to the thrombus per se. What was most interesting on scans through the chest was that there was no evidence of pulmonary emboli or infarction. A somewhat dilated azygos vein was seen, although this could in part have been related to the patient's parenchymal liver disease and portal hypertension.

References

Niehues B, Heuser L, Jansen W, Hilger HH. Noninvasive detection of intracardiac tumors by ultrasound and computed tomography. *Cardiovasc Intervent Radiol* 1983; 6:30–36.

Shin MS, Kirklin JK, Cain JB, Ho KJ. Primary angiosarcoma of the heart: CT characteristics. *AJR* 1987; 148:267–268.

Woodard PK, Sostman HD, MacFall JR, et al. Detection of pulmonary embolism: comparison of contrast-enhanced spiral CT and time-of-flight MR techniques. *J Thorac Imag* 1995; 10:59–72.

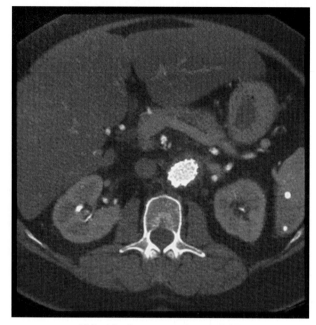

FIG. 9A. Contrast-enhanced CT

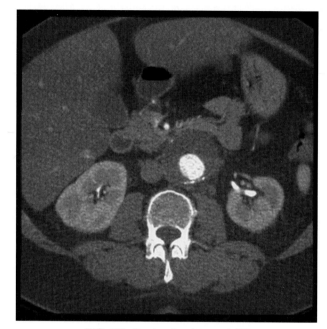

FIG. 9B. Contrast-enhanced CT

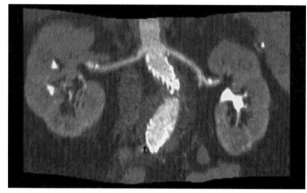

FIG. 9C. Curved reform

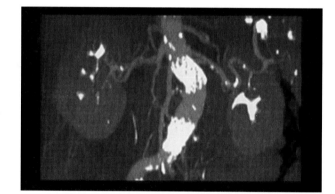

FIG. 9D. MIP

History

A patient who had undergone endoluminal stent grafting for an abdominal aortic aneurysm.

Findings

Figures 9A and B are axial scans from a three-dimensional CT angiogram following stent graft placement. Notice the high-density metallic struts of the stent in Figure 9A. There is extensive thrombus in the aneurysm on Figure 9B. Figure 9C is obtained by curved planar reformation and Figure 9D is an MIP projection. In this type of stent graft there are metallic struts superiorly and inferiorly, with mesh in between. The renal arteries are shown to be patent. The stent graft has been positioned just below the renal arteries.

Diagnosis

Endoluminal stent graft of an abdominal aortic aneurysm.

Discussion

Endoluminal stent grafting of aneurysms has revolutionized the treatment of vascular disease. Although most of the early work has been done with thoracic aortic aneurysms, owing to the high morbidity of surgery, abdominal aortic aneurysms are also amenable to endoluminal stent grafting. This patient demonstrated a very good result from the stent graft because the aneurysm was completely thrombosed and the renal and iliac arteries remained patent.

References

Balm R, Eikelboom BC, van Leeuwen MS, Noordzij J. Spiral CT-angiography of the aorta. *Eur J Vasc Surg* 1994; 8:544–551.

Semba CP, Rubin GD, Dake MD. Three-dimensional spiral CT angiography of the abdomen. *Semin Ultrasound CT MR* 1994; 15:133–138.

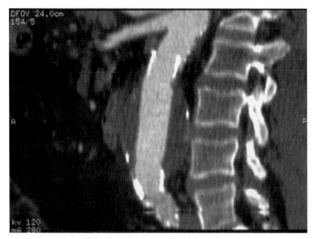

FIG. 10A. Sagittal reformation

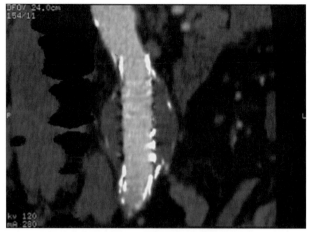

FIG. 10B. Coronal reformation

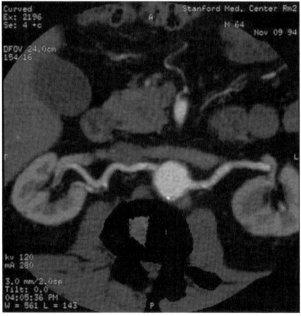

FIG. 10C. Curved reformation

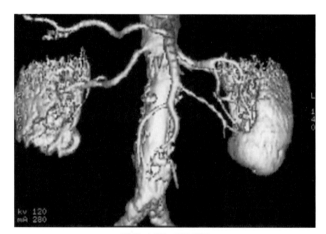

FIG. 10D. 3D CT

History

A patient who had undergone endoluminal placement of an aortic stent graft for an abdominal aortic aneurysm.

Findings

Figure 10A is a sagittal reformation of the aorta demonstrating thrombosis within the aneurysm. The metallic portions of the stent graft are seen above the aortic bifurcation and below the superior mesenteric artery. Figure 10B is a coronal reformation of the stent graft demonstrating patency of the aorta with thrombosis of the aneurysm. Figure 10C is a curved planar reformation demonstrating patency of the renal arteries. Figure 10D is a shaded-surface display demonstrating the vascular anatomy of the aorta after placement of the stent graft.

Diagnosis

Abdominal aortic aneurysm treated by endoluminal stent grafting.

Discussion

Endoluminal stent grafting is rapidly becoming the treatment of choice for a large variety of thoracoabdominal aneurysms. Three-dimensional CT angiography (CTA) (particularly using curved planar reformations) is an excellent method for following patients after stent grafting. The relationship of the stent to the lumen of the aneurysm can be determined, as well as the patency of major splanchnic vessels and the stent graft itself. Early complications, such as stent-graft leakage and intimal or thrombus formation, may be identified with CTA.

References

Dake MD; Miller DC; Semba CP; Mitchell RS; Walker PJ; Liddell RP. Transluminal placement of endovascular stent-grafts for the treatment of descending thoracic aortic aneurysms. *N Engl J Med* 1994; 331:1729–1734.

Balm R, Eikelboom BC, van Leeuwen MS, Noordzij J. Spiral CT-angiography of the aorta. *Eur J Vasc Surg* 1994; 8:544–551.

Semba CP, Rubin GD, Dake MD. Three-dimensional spiral CT angiography of the abdomen. *Semin Ultrasound CT MR* 1994; 15:133–138.

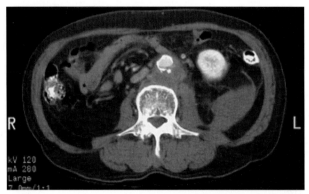

FIG. 11A. Contrast-enhanced CT

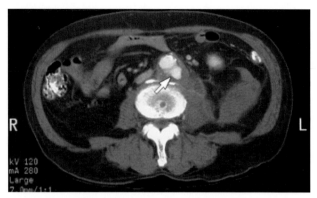

FIG. 11B. Contrast-enhanced CT

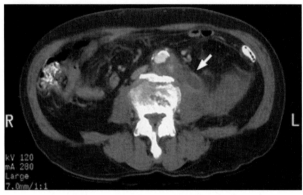

FIG. 11C. Contrast-enhanced CT

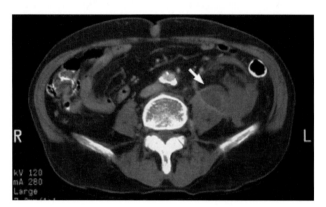

FIG. 11D. Contrast-enhanced CT

History

Acute left flank pain and falling hematocrit.

Findings

Figures 11A–D are contrast-enhanced spiral CT scans of the abdomen. Note in Figure 11B a focal protrusion along the posterolateral margin of the abdominal aorta, consistent with a penetrating ulcer (arrow). Note the psoas compartment and retroperitoneal hemorrhage (arrows, Figure 11C and D). In Figure 11A, retroaortic hemorrhage is noted displacing the aorta anteriorly.

Diagnosis

Ruptured penetrating ulcer of the abdominal aorta.

Discussion

The excellent contrast-enhancement of the aorta with spiral CT clearly demonstrates the penetrating ulcer and surrounding hemorrhage. Although relatively rare in the abdominal aorta, penetrating ulcers are not uncommon in the descending thoracic aorta and may mimic aortic dissections. Perforation with exsanguinating hemorrhage may result unless the ulcer is treated promptly. The surgical repair is often more extensive than for aortic dissections. In the future it is likely that many of these patients will be treated with endoluminal stent grafts. This patient was sent directly to surgery for aortic repair, and made an uneventful recovery.

References

Braverman AC. Penetrating atherosclerotic ulcers of the aorta. *Curr Opin Cardiol* 1994; 9:591–597.

Harris JA, Bir KG, Glover JL, Bendick JP, Shetty A, Brown OW. Penetrating atherosclerotic ulcers of the aorta. *J Vasc Surg* 1994; 19:90–98.

Kazerooni EA; Bree RL, Williams DM. Penetrating atherosclerotic ulcers of the descending thoracic aorta: evaluation with CT and distinction from aortic dissection. *Radiology* 1992; 183:759–765.

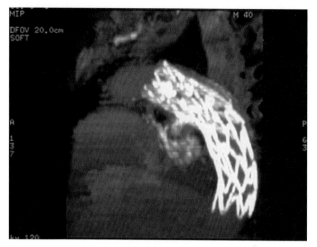

FIG. 12A. MIP

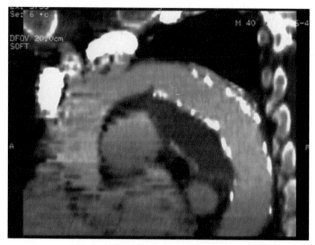

FIG. 12B. Curved reformation

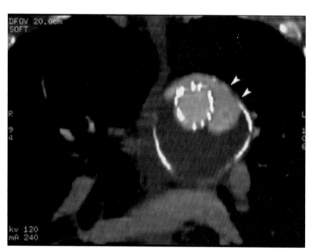

FIG. 12C. Coronal reformation

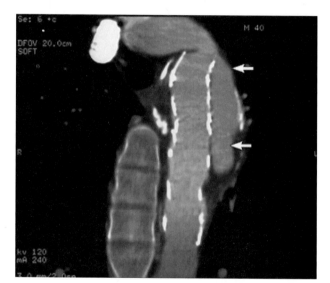

FIG. 12D. Curved reformation

History

Thoracic aortic aneurysm, status post endoluminal stent grafting.

Findings

Figures 12A–D are scans of the thoracic aorta obtained during a three-dimensional spiral CT angiogram. Figure 12A is a maximal intensity projection (MIP) demonstrating an endoluminal stent graft in the aortic arch. Figure 12B is a curved planar reformation through the aortic arch. Note the low-density thrombus within the aneurysm and contrast enhancement within the stent graft. In Figure 12C and D notice a small amount of leakage of contrast (arrows) into a portion of the aneurysm that is still patent.

Diagnosis

Endoluminal stent graft of a thoracic aortic aneurysm with persistent patency of a portion of the aneurysm.

Discussion

In this patient a small portion of the thoracic aortic aneurysm was still patent after the placement of the endoluminal stent graft. This can be due either to failure to cover the entire inflow of the aneurysm with the stent graft or to an actual tear or fenestration of the stent graft itself. The use of curved planar reformations is essential to visualize the inside of the endoluminal stent graft, since neither shaded-surface displays nor MIPs will provide intraluminal detail. Axial source images are also important to review in addition to reformations. In a number of patients, small leaks into the thoracic aneurysm following stent grafting may ultimately thrombose within a few months. If the aneurysm is still patent at 3 months, however, repeat grafting may be performed to ensure complete occlusion of the aneurysm. Alternatively, the small portion of the aneurysm that is still patent may be embolized with steel coils.

References

Balm R, Eikelboom BC, van Leeuwen MS, Noordzij J. Spiral CT-angiography of the aorta. *Eur J Vasc Surg* 1994; 8:544–551.

Semba CP, Rubin GD, Dake MD. Three-dimensional spiral CT angiography of the abdomen. *Semin Ultrasound CT MR* 1994; 15:133–138.

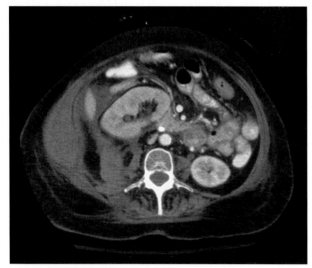

FIG. 13A. Contrast-enhanced CT

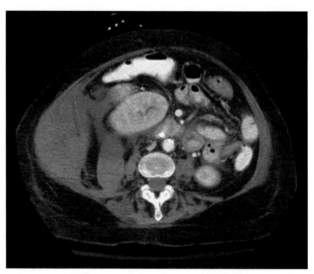

FIG. 13B. Contrast-enhanced CT

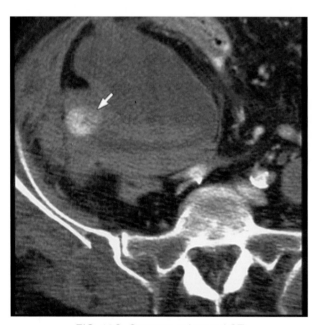

FIG. 13C. Contrast-enhanced CT

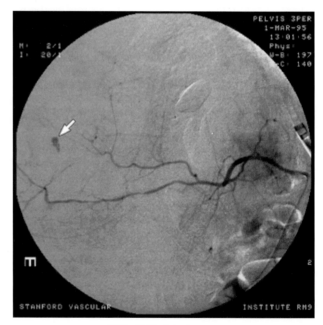

FIG. 13D. Arteriogram

History

Falling hematocrit and right flank pain. The patient is receiving anticoagulant therapy for atrial fibrillation.

Findings

Figures 13A and B are contrast-enhanced spiral CT scans at the level of the kidney, demonstrating a large retroperitoneal hematoma displacing the right kidney toward the midline. Figure 13C is a magnified image of the right iliac fossa demonstrating a punctate focus of extremely high attenuation within a large hematoma (arrow). This area is consistent with active arterial extravasation. Figure 13D is a selective right lumbar arteriogram demonstrating a focal area of arterial extravasation (arrow).

Diagnosis

Active retroperitoneal arterial extravasation diagnosed with spiral CT.

Discussion

The identification and localization of active arterial extravasation related to excessive anticoagulation was critical in managing this patient. Because of the retroperitoneal location of the extravasation in the iliac fossa, the likelihood of a lumbar artery hemorrhage was strongly entertained, and the patient was taken directly to angiography. Following a midstream aortogram and selective catheterization of the lumbar arteries, a bleeding lumbar vessel was identified and selectively embolized.

Patients with lumbar artery hemorrhage are often difficult to approach surgically because identification of the lumbar arteries, in the presence of a large retroperitoneal hematoma, is hazardous and time consuming. This patient made an uneventful recovery following embolization, despite extensive blood loss. Areas of active arterial extravasation are almost always embedded within large hematomas. They are isodense with major arterial structures, and are often irregular in their configuration. The detection of active arterial extravasation generally indicates the need for urgent surgery or embolization. Conservative therapy is not warranted in these patients.

References

Jeffrey RB Jr, Cardoza JD, Olcott EW. Detection of active intraabdominal arterial hemorrhage: value of dynamic contrast-enhanced CT. *AJR* 1991; 156:725–729.

O'Sullivan G, Williams M, Hughes PM. Mesenteric arterial rupture following blunt abdominal trauma: demonstration by computed tomography (Letter). *Br J Radiol* 1994; 67:1143–1144.

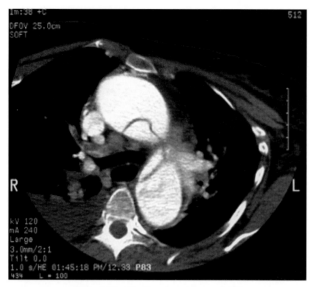

FIG. 14A. Contrast-enhanced CT

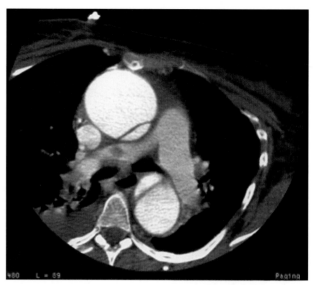

FIG. 14B. Contrast-enhanced CT

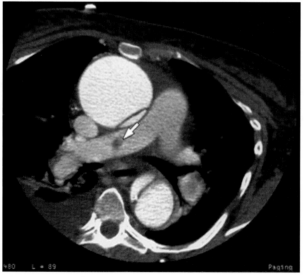

FIG. 14C. Contrast-enhanced CT

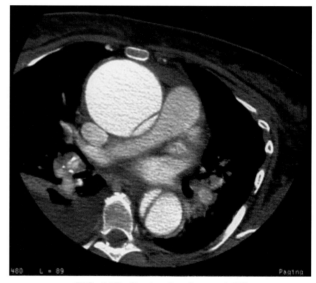

FIG. 14D. Contrast-enhanced CT

History

Crushing chest pain. Rule out aortic dissection.

Findings

Figures 14A–D are spiral CT scans of the mediastinum performed with intravenous contrast enhancement. There is an aneurysm of the ascending aorta. Note also the excellent depiction of a type A dissection involving both the ascending and descending thoracic aorta. In Figure 14A and C filling defects are seen in the pulmonary arteries, consistent with a pulmonary embolus (arrow). Notice the large right pleural effusion.

Diagnosis

Type A aortic dissection, pulmonary embolism, and aneurysm of the ascending aorta.

Discussion

Transesophageal sonography is often the first diagnostic study in patients with suggested aortic dissection. The pulmonary embolism evident in this case would not have been confirmed by the transesophageal technique. On CT the intimal flap was clearly noted from the top of the arch to extend into the upper abdomen. Other views of the neck showed extension into the great vessels as well. Compared to MRI, spiral CT has the advantage of speed, since most of these studies take less than 5 to 10 minutes to perform. Although the reconstruction time may be longer, depending upon the number of slices, the examination is still much faster than MRI. Spiral CT may be a useful alternative to lung scanning for pulmonary emboli. It is as yet unproven in the diagnosis of small peripheral emboli.

References

Blum AG, Delfau F, Grignon B, et al. Spiral-computed tomography versus pulmonary angiography in the diagnosis of acute massive pulmonary embolism. *Am J Cardiol* 1994; 74:96–98.

Matsumoto AHJ, Tegtmeyer CJ. Contemporary diagnostic approaches to acute pulmonary emboli. *Radiol Clin North Am* 1995; 33:167–183.

Remy-Jardin M, Remy J, Wattinne L, Giraud F. Central pulmonary thromboembolism: diagnosis with spiral volumetric CT with the single-breath-hold technique—comparison with pulmonary angiography. *Radiology* 1992; 185:381–387.

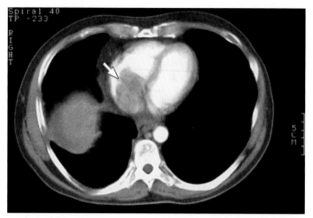

FIG. 15A. Contrast-enhanced CT

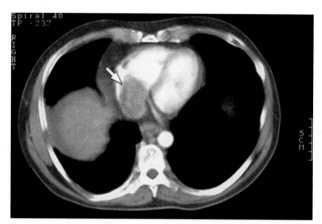

FIG. 15B. Contrast-enhanced CT

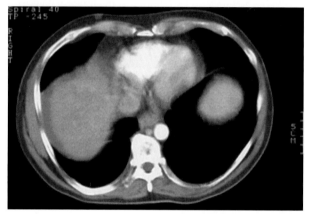

FIG. 15C. Contrast-enhanced CT

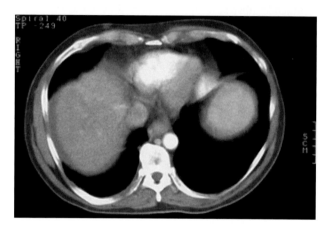

FIG. 15D. Contrast-enhanced CT

History

A 63-year-old male with a clinical history suggesting a possible hepatoma. The CT scan was done for evaluation.

Findings

A spiral CT scan demonstrates a filling defect representing a mass in the right atrium. The mass appears to be partially lobulated and extends into the inferior vena cava.

Diagnosis

Hepatoma with extension into the inferior vena cava and right atrium.

Discussion

Spiral CT is an excellent method for detecting the presence of hepatocellular carcinoma and determining its extent. Spiral CT coupled with multiplanar and three-dimensional reconstruction can be used for preoperative surgical planning.

This case demonstrates the value of spiral CT in determining the extent of disease. There is a mass present in the right atrium, which is actually tumor extension from hepatoma via the inferior vena cava. Intracardiac masses are typically evaluated by echocardiography or MRI. However, echocardiography does have problems in certain areas, including cases of right atrial tumors that arise from intraabdominal processes. MRI is excellent in defining these processes.

A mass within the right atrium can be a malignant or benign tumor. These tumors can be primary or metastatic. Primary tumors of the heart and pericardium are found in less than 0.1% of autopsy series. Of these, two-thirds are benign. The most common benign tumor involving the atrium is a myxoma, which tends to be more common in the left atrium than the right.

In our experience, tumor extension from the abdomen is a more common cause of right atrial thrombus. Tumors that can extend off the inferior vena cava include hepatoma, renal-cell carcinoma, and adrenal cancer. Tumors primary to the inferior vena cava, such as inferior vena cava (IVC) sarcoma, can also extend upward. IVC sarcomas tend to be very vascular and may extend over long distances, but they can usually be distinguished from extension of a hepatoma or renal-cell carcinoma, which are typically not hypervascular on CT scanning.

References

Gross BH, Glazer GM, Francis IR. CT of intracardiac and intrapericardial masses. *AJR* 1983; 140:903–907.

Honda H, Ochiai K, Adachi E, et al. Hepatocellular carcinoma: correlation of CT, angiographic, and histopathologic findings. *Radiology* 1993; 189:857–862.

Woodhouse CE, Ney DR, Sitzmann JV, Fishman EK. Spiral computed tomography arterial portography with three-dimensional volumetric rendering for oncologic surgery planning. *Invest Radiol* 1995; 29:1031–1037.

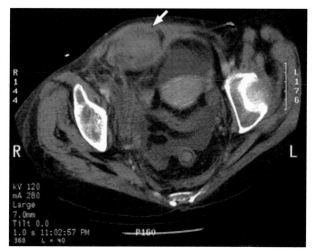

FIG. 16A. Contrast-enhanced CT

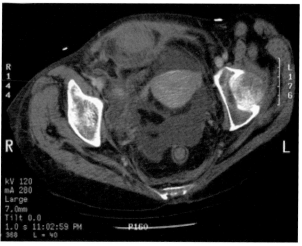

FIG. 16B. Contrast-enhanced CT

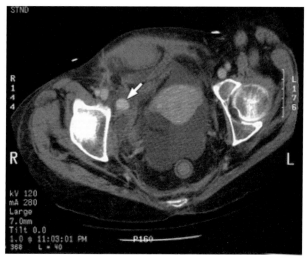

FIG. 16C. Contrast-enhanced CT

History

Falling hematocrit after intravenous anticoagulation for coronary artery stent.

Findings

Figures 16A–C are spiral CT scans of the pelvis demonstrating a large extraperitoneal hematoma involving the right pelvic side wall and rectus sheath (arrow). In Figure 16C, notice a focus of active arterial extravasation, adjacent to the obturator internis muscle, that is isodense with the external iliac artery (arrow).

Diagnosis

Active arterial extravasation due to excessive anticoagulation.

Discussion

The anatomic site of the patient's active arterial extravasation was clearly depicted on the spiral CT scan of the pelvis. Patients with hematomas without arterial extravasation may be treated conservatively with correction of coagulation parameters. However, in the presence of active arterial extravasation, either immediate surgery or embolization is required to stop the bleeding. In this patient, emergency pelvic surgery was performed, which identified active arterial extravasation from branches of the external iliac artery. The hematoma in the right rectus sheath was probably also related to spontaneous hemorrhage, from a branch of the inferior epigastric artery.

References

Jeffrey RB Jr, Cardoza JD, Olcott EW. Detection of active intraabdominal arterial hemorrhage: value of dynamic contrast-enhanced CT. *AJR* 1991; 156:725–729.

O'Sullivan G, Williams M, Hughes PM. Mesenteric arterial rupture following blunt abdominal trauma: demonstration by computed tomography (letter). *Br J Radiol* 1994; 67:1143–1144.

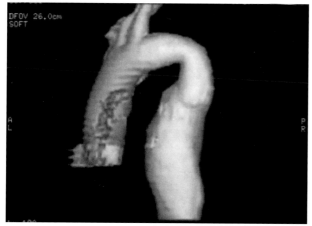

FIG. 17A. 3D CT

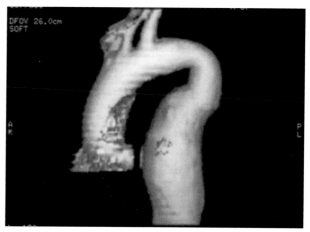

FIG. 17B. 3D CT

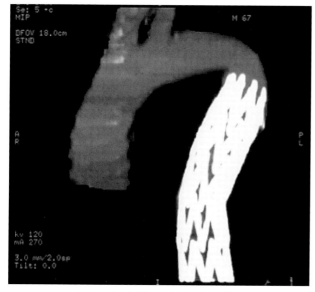

FIG. 17C. MIP post stent grafting

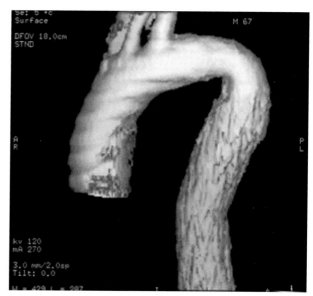

FIG. 17D. Shaded-surface display post stent grafting

History

Enlarging thoracic aortic aneurysm on chest x-ray.

Findings

Figures 17A and B are shaded-surface display images from a three-dimensional spiral CT angiogram. Note the large aneurysm involving the descending thoracic aorta. Figures 17C and D are MIP and shaded-surface display images obtained after placement of an endoluminal stent graft. Note the lack of contrast enhancement of the aneurysm.

Diagnosis

Descending thoracic aortic aneurysm treated by endovascular stent grafting.

Discussion

Surgical resection of descending thoracic aortic aneurysms is associated with a high frequency of morbidity and mortality. The development of endovascular techniques with stent grafts is likely to play a major role in the management of these patients. Three-dimensional CT angiography is the ideal technique for evaluating these patients both before and after stent-graft placement. Magnetic resonance angiography is not feasible in patients with indwelling metallic devices. In this patient the endoluminal stent graft was successful in occluding the aneurysm. The follow-up CT angiogram demonstrated no flow within the peripheral portion of the aneurysm.

References

Balm R, Eikelboom BC, van Leeuwen MS, Noordzij J. Spiral CT-angiography of the aorta. *Eur J Vasc Surg* 1994; 8:544–551.

Dake MD, Miller DC, Semba CP, Mitchell RS, Walker PJ, Liddell RP. Transluminal placement of endovascular stent-grafts for the treatment of descending thoracic aortic aneurysms. *N Engl J Med* 1994; 331:1729–1734.

Semba CP, Rubin GD, Dake MD. Three-dimensional spiral CT angiography of the abdomen. *Semin Ultrasound CT MR* 1994; 15:133–138.

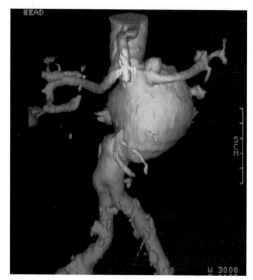

FIG. 18A. 3D CT

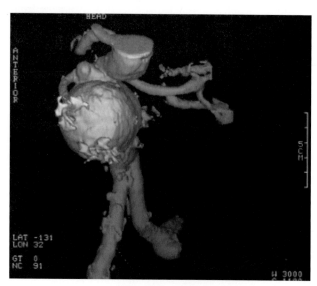

FIG. 18B. 3D CT

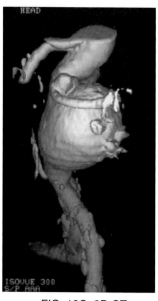

FIG. 18C. 3D CT

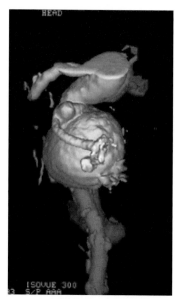

FIG. 18D. 3D CT

History

A patient who had undergone aortobifemoral bypass surgery. Enlarging abdominal aortic aneurysm on sonography.

Findings

Figure 18A–D are shaded-surface displays obtained from a three-dimensional spiral CT angiogram. The aortobifemoral bypass is patent. A large saccular abdominal aortic aneurysm is identified involving the renal arteries. There is saccular extension of the aneurysm into the proximal left renal artery. There is a single right renal artery, but no definable infrarenal neck to the aneurysm.

Diagnosis

Saccular aneurysm of the abdominal aorta involving the left renal artery.

Discussion

The preoperative evaluation of the abdominal aorta prior to surgery for aneurysm must define the relationship of the aneurysm to the visceral vessels, the renal arteries, and the iliac bifurcation. More than 95% of abdominal aortic aneurysms are infrarenal and do not involve the renal arteries. However, involvement of the renal arteries often necessitates surgical reimplantation, and is of critical importance to determine preoperatively. In this patient there was clear involvement of the left renal artery, which had to be reimplanted at surgery. A supraceliac aortic clamp was used, which has a higher rate of morbidity because of associated renal ischemia.

References

Balm R, Eikelboom BC, van Leeuwen MS, Noordzij J. Spiral CT-angiography of the aorta. *Eur J Vasc Surg* 1994; 8:544–551.

Semba CP, Rubin GD, Dake MD. Three-dimensional spiral CT angiography of the abdomen. *Semin Ultrasound CT MR* 1994; 15:133–138.

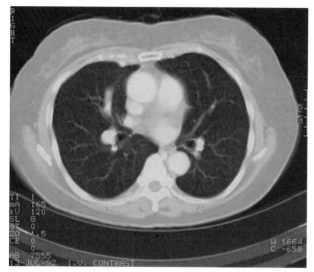

FIG. 19A. Contrast-enhanced CT

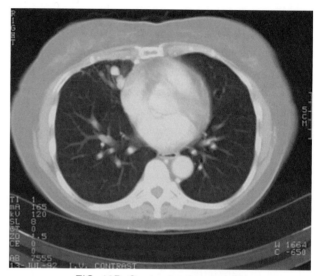

FIG. 19B. Contrast-enhanced CT

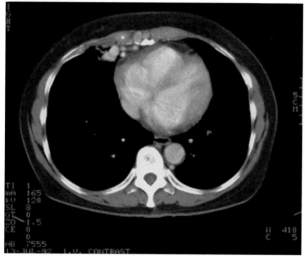

FIG. 19C. Contrast-enhanced CT

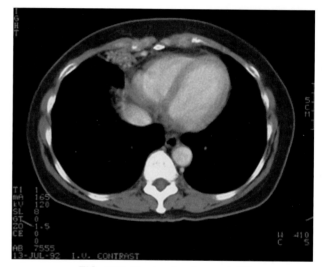

FIG. 19D. Contrast-enhanced CT

History

A 65-year-old female who presented with a right-lower-lung lesion on chest x-ray.

Findings

A spiral CT scan demonstrates a weblike configuration of vessels near the right cardiophrenic angle, which corresponds to the area of the mass seen on the chest radiograph. More cranial scans demonstrate a large feeding vessel extending toward the vascular network.

Diagnosis

Pulmonary arteriovenous malformation simulating a pulmonary mass.

Discussion

Arteriovenous malformations can simulate solitary lung masses on routine chest radiographs. However, on spiral CT, it is fairly easy to recognize them by demonstrating both the large feeding vessel and draining vessels. As in this case, the lesions may be serpiginous. They are optimally defined with contrast enhancement, but because of their configuration can be recognized without contrast enhancement.

There have been several articles in the CT literature describing the role of three-dimensional imaging for the evaluation of arteriovenous malformations. Remy et al. reviewed 37 pulmonary arteriovenous malformations with both spiral CT and pulmonary angiography. The authors used single-threshold shaded-surface displays and evaluated their patients without injection of contrast material. A reliable analysis of the architecture of 28 pulmonary arteriovenous mal-

formations (75%) was provided by three-dimensional reconstructions alone. Combining interpretation of the three-dimensional reconstructions with the transaxial images led to accurate evaluation in 35 of the pulmonary arteriovenous malformations (94%). The authors concluded that unenhanced three-dimensional spiral CT is a reliable noninvasive tool for the pretreatment evaluation of pulmonary venous malformations.

Based on the authors' results, we agree that this is an excellent technique to use. However, we feel that contrast enhancement can be valuable in defining the full extent of any unusual vascular components to arteriovenous malformations. We recommend a non-contrast-enhanced spiral CT followed by an enhanced spiral CT scan to optimize lesion evaluation.

References

Napel S, Marks MP, Rubin GD, et al. CT angiography with spiral CT and maximum intensity projection. *Radiology* 1992; 185:607–610.

Remy J, Remy-Jardin M, Giraud F, Wattinne L. Angioarchitecture of pulmonary arteriovenous malformations: clinical utility of three-dimensional helical CT. *Radiology* 1994; 191:657–664.

Remy J, Remy-Jardin M, Wattinne L, Defontaines C. Pulmonary arteriovenous malformations: evaluation with CT of the chest before and after treatment. *Radiology* 1992; 182:809–816.

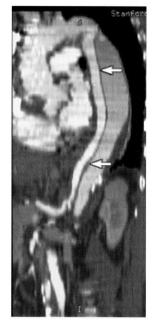

FIG. 20A. Sagittal reformation CT

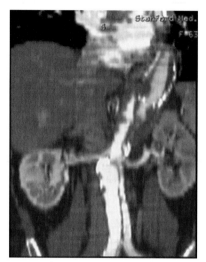

FIG. 20B. Coronal reformation CT

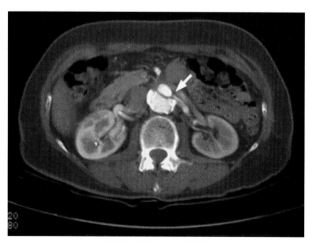

FIG. 20C. Axial CT

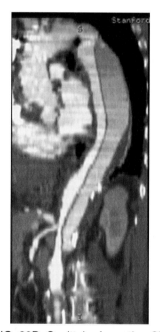

FIG. 20D. Sagittal reformation CT

History

Severe chest and back pain. Rule out aortic dissection.

Findings

Figures 20A is a sagittal curved planar reformation of a spiral CT angiogram demonstrating an intimal flap originating distal to the left subclavian artery and extending into the upper abdomen (arrow). Figure 20B demonstrates that the flap extends to the level of the aortic bifurcation. Figure 20C is an axial image taken from the same data set and clearly demonstrating extension of the internal flap into the left renal artery (arrow). Figure 20D is another sagittal view of the dissection, demonstrating that the superior mesentery artery originates from the true lumen.

Diagnosis

Extensive thoracoabdominal aortic dissection.

Discussion

MRI and transesophageal echocardiography (TEE) are often the primary screening modalities for evaluating patients with suspected aortic dissections. However, spiral CT may also be quite useful, and has a number of imaging advantages. Chief among these are speed and ease of interpretation. Magnetic resonance imaging (MRI), although able to quantitate flow and to generate dynamic images with phase-contrast gradient echographic techniques, often takes 1 hour to perform. Spiral CT can be performed within 10–15 minutes and the data set can be edited to perform a variety of reformations. In this patient, the curved planar reformations were quite helpful in displaying the entire extent of the dissection and viewing the takeoff of visceral vessels from either the true or false lumen. However, it should be pointed out that axial source images are often best for viewing the extension of dissection flaps into the renal arteries, as is demonstrated nicely in Figure 20C.

References

Alfrey EJ, Rubin GD, Kuo PC, et al. The use of spiral computed tomography in the evaluation of living donors for kidney transplantation. *Transplantation* 1995; 59:4:643–645.

Mell MW, Alfrey EJ, Rubin GD, Scandling JD, Jeffrey RB Jr, Dafoe DC. Use of spiral computed tomography in the diagnosis of transplant renal stenosis. *Transplantation* 1994; 57:746–779.

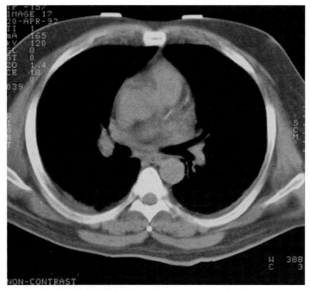

FIG. 21A. Non-contrast–enhanced CT

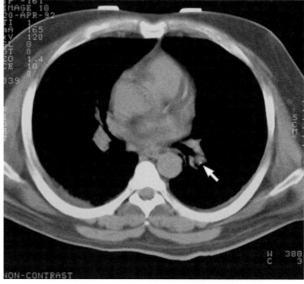

FIG. 21B. Non-contrast–enhanced CT

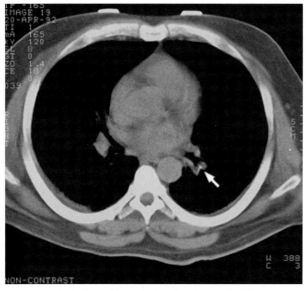

FIG. 21C. Non-contrast–enhanced CT

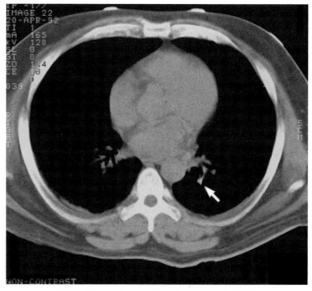

FIG. 21D. Non-contrast–enhanced CT

History

A 47-year-old male who presented to an outside hospital with severe chest pain and findings corresponding to myocardial infarction. The patient had coronary angiography, which showed three-vessel disease. The patient then underwent successful percutaneous transluminal angioplasty (PTCA) of the circumflex vessels. At the time of angioplasty, foreign objects were observed in the left pulmonary artery, possibly representing guidewires. The patient was sent for CT for further evaluation.

Findings

A spiral CT scan with narrow interscan collimation demonstrates an opaque radiodensity in the left main pulmonary artery, consistent with findings made on fluoroscopy.

Diagnosis

Broken catheter in the left pulmonary artery.

Discussion

The spiral CT findings were compatible with a probable broken catheter. The patient was sent to the cardiovascular laboratory where the broken catheter was successfully retrieved. The broken component was shown to be the Teflon sheath of the catheter.

Complications related to catheter breakage are rare. However, when they do occur, recent interventional procedural developments allow the cardiovascular radiologist to remove the misplaced or broken foreign bodies before they can cause any further complication. In the present case, a small catheter was removed from the left pulmonary artery. Spiral CT was helpful in this case by specifically revealing and localizing the foreign body. In addition, based on the CT attenuation, it was assumed that the findings were due to a catheter and not to a thrombus in the vessel.

References

Godwin JD, Chen JTT. Thoracic venous anatomy. *AJR* 1986; 147:674–684.
O'Callaghan JP, Heitzman ER, Somogyi JW, Spirt BA. CT evaluation of pulmonary artery size. *J Comput Assist Tomogr* 1982; 6(1):101–104.

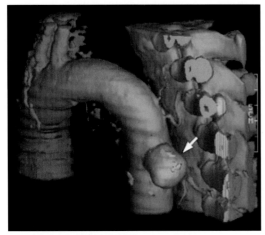

FIG. 22A. Shaded-surface display CT

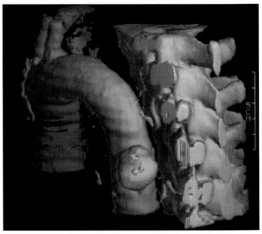

FIG. 22B. Shaded-surface display CT

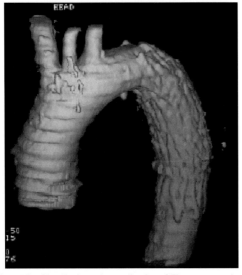

FIG. 22C. Shaded-surface display CT post stenting

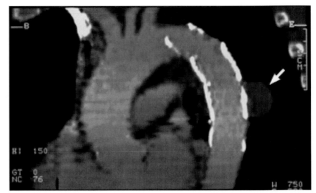

FIG. 22D. Curved plane reformation

History

Known thoracic aortic aneurysm.

Findings

Figures 22A and B are shaded-surface displays obtained from a three-dimensional spiral CT angiogram of the thoracic aorta. Note the saccular aneurysm (arrow), approximately 2 cm in size, extending from the descending thoracic aorta. Figure 22C is a shaded-surface display after the insertion of an endoluminal stent graft. Note the lack of filling of the aneurysm. Figure 22D is a curved planar reformation demonstrating a patent lumen off the stent graft and thrombosis within the aneurysm (arrow).

Diagnosis

Saccular aneurysm of the thoracic aorta, occluded with an endoluminal stent graft.

Discussion

The shaded surface display images clearly demonstrated the focal aneurysm of the descending thoracic aorta. The great vessels were not involved and there was no evidence of aortic dissection. The treatment of choice for a focal aneurysm of the descending thoracic aorta is now endoluminal stent grafting. This can be done with a minimum of morbidity and expense. The stent graft is placed above and below the aneurysm, creating a neointima and thus occluding the aneurysm. Spiral CT angiography is the imaging technique of choice for evaluating the aorta after stent grafting.

References

Balm R, Eikelboom BC, van Leeuwen MS, Noordzij J. Spiral CT-angiography of the aorta. *Eur J Vasc Surg* 1994; 8:544–551.

Semba CP, Rubin GD, Dake MD. Three-dimensional spiral CT angiography of the abdomen. *Semin Ultrasound CT MR* 1994; 15:133–138.

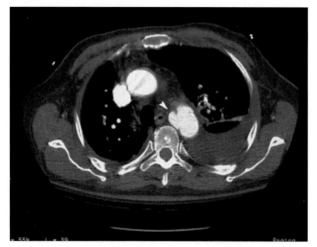

FIG. 23A. Contrast-enhanced CT

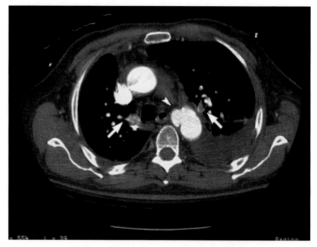

FIG. 23B. Contrast-enhanced CT

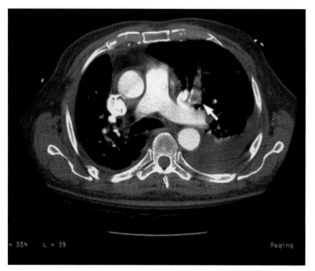

FIG. 23C. Contrast-enhanced CT

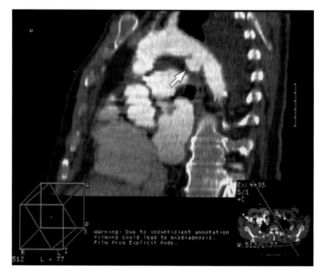

FIG. 23D. Sagittal reformation

History

A 71-year-old male with a widened mediastinum on chest x-ray following blunt chest trauma.

Findings

Figure 23A–C are contrast-enhanced spiral CT scans of the thorax. Note the large left pleural effusion and the pseudoaneurysm of the thoracic aorta in the region of the ligamentum arteriosum (arrowhead). Figure 23B and C demonstrate filling defects in the left pulmonary arteries consistent with pulmonary emboli (arrows). Figure 23D is a sagittal reformation of the aortic arch demonstrating the aortic rupture with pseu-

doaneurysm formation (arrow). Figure 23E and F were obtained after an endoluminal stent graft was placed percutaneously into the transverse portion of the thoracic aortic arch. In addition, a metallic stent was placed in the left subclavian artery. Note that there is no filling of the pseudoaneurysm, which is now occluded.

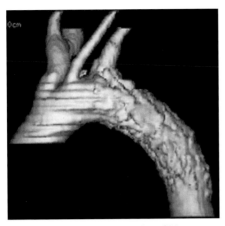

FIG. 23E. Shaded-surface display CT post stenting

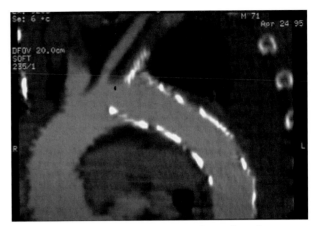

FIG. 23F. Curved-planar reformation of
aortic arch post stenting

Diagnosis

Traumatic rupture of the thoracic aorta treated by endoluminal stent grafting. Pulmonary emboli.

Discussion

Traumatic rupture of the aorta causes immediate fatality in nearly 90% of patients. Of the 10% of patients that survive the immediate trauma, approximately 50% will die within the first 24 hours unless there is prompt surgical treatment. Angiography has traditionally been performed in all patients with a wide mediastinum after blunt closed-chest trauma. Spiral CT in patients who are able to cooperate and hold their breath may be a useful alternative in these patients.

Endoluminal stent grafting offers a novel approach to treating this lesion. This patient was at high risk from surgery because of the associated pulmonary emboli diagnosed by spiral CT. After it was inserted, the endoluminal stent graft in the aortic arch covered a portion of the subclavian artery. Therefore, a metallic stent was placed in the origin of the subclavian artery to ensure its patency. At present, the diagnostic accuracy of CT for detecting traumatic rupture of the aorta is unknown. One potential value of CT is to assess the mediastinum for blood. A normal CT virtually excludes the diagnosis of aortic rupture. Had angiography been performed alone, pulmonary emboli would not have been diagnosed in this case.

References

Durham RM, Zuckerman D, Wolverson M, et al. Computed tomography as a screening exam in patients with suspected blunt aortic injury. *Ann Surg* 1994; 220:699–704.

Fisher RG, Chasen MH, Lamki N. Diagnosis of injuries of the aorta and brachiocephalic arteries caused by blunt chest trauma: CT vs aortography. *AJR* 1994; 162:1047–1052.

Hughes JP, Ruttley MS, Musumeci F. Case report: traumatic aortic rupture: demonstration by magnetic resonance imaging. *Br J Radiol* 1994; 67:1264–1267.

Wilson D, Voystock JF, Sariego J, Kerstein MD. Role of computed tomography scan in evaluating the widened mediastinum. *Am Surg* 1994; 60:421–423.

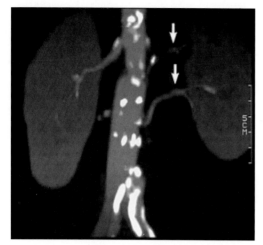

FIG. 24A. MIP

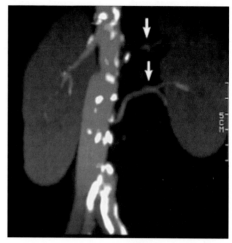

FIG. 24B. MIP

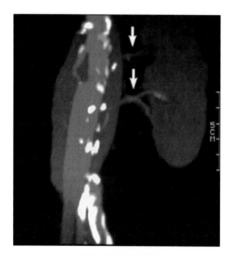

FIG. 24C. MIP

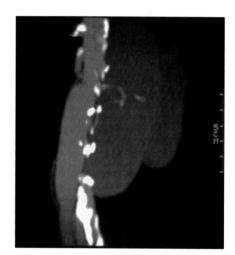

FIG. 24D. MIP

History

Status post aortobifemoral bypass with reimplantation of the left renal arteries.

Findings

Figures 24A–D are maximum intensity projections (MIP) from a three-dimensional CT angiogram. Note that the aortobifemoral graft is patent and that the two renal arteries on the left are patent (arrows). The native renal artery on the right is also well visualized. The native distal aorta is identified on the more lateral views (Figure 23C and D). The kidneys demonstrate symmetric nephrograms without evidence of infarction.

Diagnosis

Status post-aortobifemoral graft. Reimplanted left renal arteries.

Discussion

Three-dimensional CT angiography is an excellent technique for evaluating post-operative patients following complicated graft surgery. In this patient, both upper- and lower-pole left renal arteries were reimplanted at the time of aneurysm resection and bifemoral grafting. The MIP clearly demonstrate that these vessels are patent and that there are symmetric nephrograms. Calcifications can clearly be seen on the MIP which, unlike the shaded-surface displays, allows differentiation for enhancing lumens, other vessels, intramural thrombus, and calcifications.

References

Balm R, Eikelboom BC, van Leeuwen MS, Noordzij J. Spiral CT-angiography of the aorta. *Eur J Vasc Surg* 1994; 8:544–551.

Semba CP, Rubin GD, Dake MD. Three-dimensional spiral CT angiography of the abdomen. *Semin Ultrasound CT MR* 1994; 15:133–138.

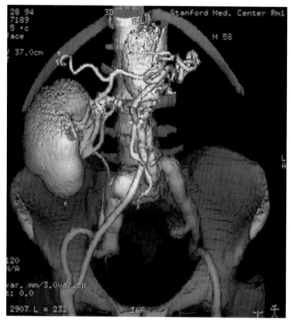

FIG. 25A. 3D CT

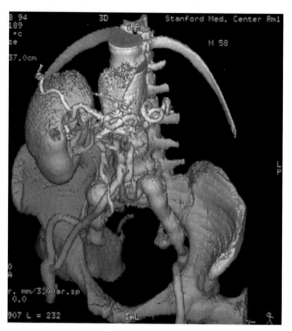

FIG. 25B. 3D CT

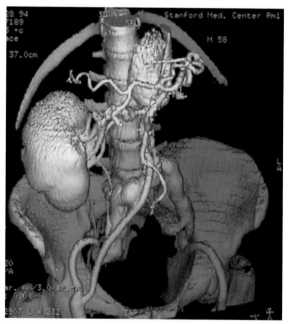

FIG. 25C. 3D CT

History

Status post-aortobifemoral bypass graft.

Findings

Figures 25A–C are shaded-surface displays from a three-dimensional CT angiogram of the aortoiliac circulation. Notice that there is no visualization of the left kidney, with compensatory hypertrophy of the spare right kidney. A graft is seen from the aorta to the right common femoral artery on the right. The left limb of the bypass graft is occluded. There is aneurysmal dilation of both the native right and left common arteries. The left limb of the graft is not visualized.

Diagnosis

Occlusion of the left renal artery and left limb of an aortobifemoral graft.

Discussion

The shaded-surface display in this patient identified lack of filling of the left limb of the bifemoral graft and the aneurysms involving both common iliac arteries. The skeletal structures are still evident, and could have been subtracted if desired. Shaded-surface displays can often be done quite rapidly as compared to other forms of three-dimensional editing. They are often useful for demonstrating vascular patency, but they are inadequate for demonstrating intraluminal thrombus, calcification, and intraluminal patency of stents or stent grafts.

References

Balm R, Eikelboom BC, van Leeuwen MS, Noordzij J. Spiral CT-angiography of the aorta. *Eur J Vasc Surg* 1994; 8:544–551.

Semba CP, Rubin GD, Dake MD. Three-dimensional spiral CT angiography of the abdomen. *Semin Ultrasound CT MR* 1994; 15:133–138.

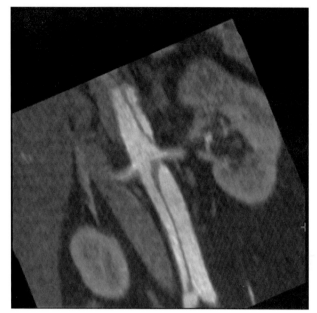

FIG. 26A. Coronal reformation

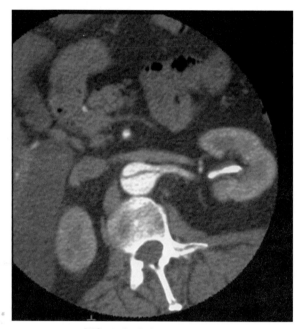

FIG. 26B. Axial reformation

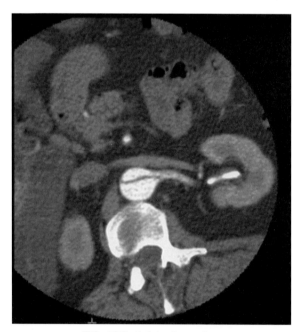

FIG. 26C. Axial reformation

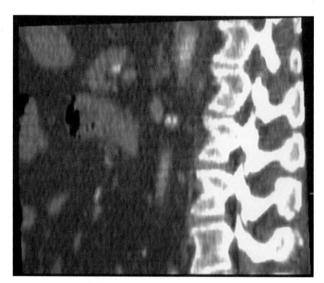

FIG. 26D. Sagittal reformation

History

Known thoracic aortic dissection. Rule out extension into the abdominal aorta.

Findings

Figure 26A and D are curved planar reformations of the abdominal aorta obtained from a three-dimensional CT angiogram. Notice the clear depiction of the intimal flap in Figure 26A–C, involving the supra- and intrarenal aorta. In Figure 26B and C notice the extension of the intimal flap into the left renal artery. However, the left kidney appears well perfused. Figure 26D is a sagittal reconstruction along the plane of the left renal artery, clearly demonstrating the intimal flap separating the true and false lumen that extends into the proximal left renal artery.

Diagnosis

Aortic dissection with extension into the left renal artery.

Discussion

The main value of the CT angiogram (CTA) in this case was the clear demonstration of the intimal flap of the aortic dissection extending into the left renal artery. The excellent spatial resolution of CTA can be quite valuable in addressing specific anatomic questions about the extent of a dissection. Dissections involving the renal artery may result in infarction, ischemia, and/or hypertension. Treatment options include surgery and endoluminal stenting.

References

Balm R, Eikelboom BC, van Leeuwen MS, Noordzij J. Spiral CT-angiography of the aorta. *Eur J Vasc Surg* 1994; 8:544–551.

Semba CP, Rubin GD, Dake MD. Three-dimensional spiral CT angiography of the abdomen. *Semin Ultrasound CT MR* 1994; 15:133–138.

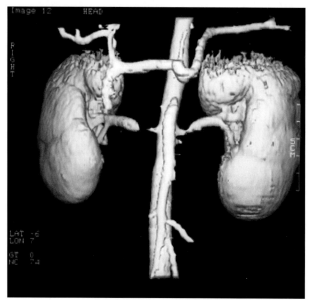

FIG. 27A. 3D CT

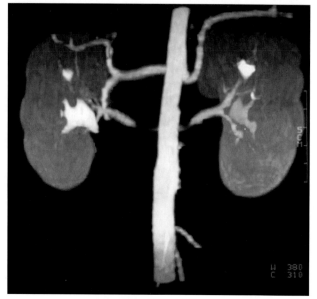

FIG. 27B. MIP

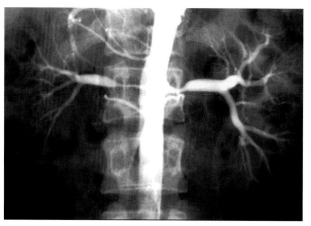

FIG. 27C. aortogram

History

A 19-year-old female with hypertension. Rule out renal artery stenosis.

Findings

Figures 27A and B are scans obtained from a three-dimensional spiral CT angiogram of the renal arteries. Figure 27A is a shaded-surface display demonstrating bilateral renal artery stenosis, greater on the right than on the left. Figure 27B is a maximal intensity projection (MIP) confirming the bilateral renal artery stenosis. Figure 27C is a film obtained from a midstream aortogram confirming the bilateral renal artery stenosis.

Diagnosis

Bilateral renal artery stenosis.

Discussion

There are several important technical factors to keep in mind when performing three-dimensional CT angiography of the renal arteries. It is important to have the patient produce a reliable breathhold and to time the peak of the bolus of contrast medium by doing a low volume (15-20 ml) test injection imaging the aorta above the level of the renal arteries. Generally, a rapid bolus of 4 to 5 ml/sec must be administered for a total of 120 to 150 ml of contrast. Because of the rapid rate of injection, nonionic contrast enhancement is essential. Three-millimeter collinated scans are obtained with a pitch of 1.5. The data set is then reconstructed with a small field of view (20 to 25 cm) at 2 mm. Shaded-surface display, maximum intensity projections (MIP), and curved-planar reformations may be necessary in individual cases. Overall, MIP projection appears to be most valuable for identifying renal-artery stenosis.

(Figure 27A–C are used by permission, Rubin et al., Radiology 1994.)

References

Balm R, Eikelboom BC, van Leeuwen MS, Noordzij J. Spiral CT-angiography of the aorta. *Eur J Vasc Surg* 1994; 8:544–551.

Rubin GD, Dake MD, Napel S, Jeffrey RB Jr, McDonnell CH, Sommer FG, Wexler L, Williams DM. Spiral CT of renal artery stenosis: comparison of three-dimensional rendering techniques. *Radiology* 1994; 190:181–189.

Semba CP, Rubin GD, Dake MD. Three-dimensional spiral CT angiography of the abdomen. *Semin Ultrasound CT MR* 1994; 15:133–138.

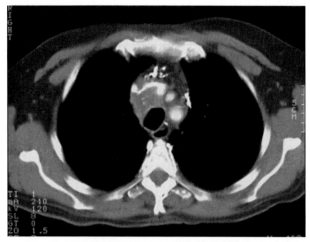

FIG. 28A. Contrast-enhanced CT

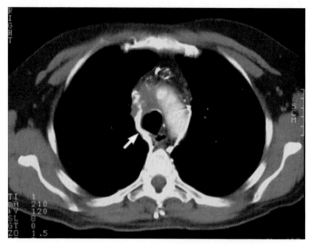

FIG. 28B. Contrast-enhanced CT

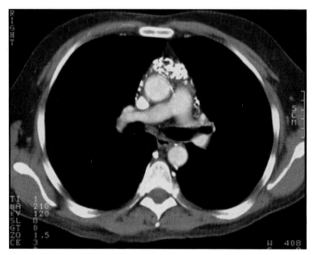

FIG. 28C. Contrast-enhanced CT

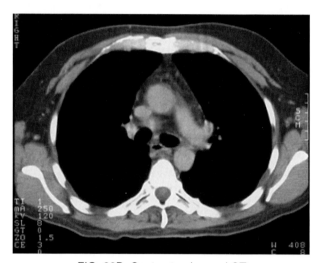

FIG. 28D. Contrast-enhanced CT

History

A 50-year-old male with a history of small-cell lung cancer. The study was done to evaluate for tumor extent following therapy.

Findings

A spiral CT scan demonstrates a tumor in the right pretracheal space with extension to and encasement of the left innominate vein near its entry into the superior vena cava. Dilated azygos (arrow) and intercostal veins are seen, as well as increased-density structures in the anterior mediastinum. A delayed CT scan was obtained, which shows that the areas of increased attenuation on the initial study are gone and were collateral vessels.

Diagnosis

Superior vena cava obstruction syndrome with anterior mediastinal collaterals.

Discussion

Superior vena cava (SVC) syndrome is the consequence of compression or obstruction of the superior vena cava by a variety of malignant or benign lesions including mediastinal masses or nodes (i.e., lung cancer, lymphoma, thymoma), fibrosing mediastinitis (i.e., due to histoplasmosis), indwelling venous catheters, or hypercoagulability states. Signs of the SVC syndrome may be detected on CT scans before the syndrome is clinically recognized by the referring physician or by the patient. Prompt diagnosis and early intervention may be critical in helping to prevent the full-blown syndrome and its possible consequences. In one study of 16 patients with CT-defined SVC syndrome, 11 of the cases were unrecognized prior to CT scanning.

Collateral pathways are the key to the early diagnosis and understanding of the SVC syndrome. Once flow to the SVC is obstructed or severely compromised, the common collateral channels seen on CT are the internal mammary vein, the azygos/hemiazygos complex, the intercostal veins, and chest-wall veins. Mediastinal veins may also be seen, although less commonly in our experience.

This case is especially interesting because of the vascularity and extent of the anterior mediastinal collaterals. In fact, at first glance they appear to be calcifications in lymph nodes, due either to granulomatous disease or to radiated lymph nodes. A delayed scan shows this to not be the case. It is interesting how on the delayed scan there is no real appreciation of dilated collateral vessels in the anterior mediastinum.

The reason for the excellent opacification of these collaterals was the use of spiral CT coupled with a rapid bolus injection of contrast medium. By scanning between 40 and 60 seconds after the initiation of injection, one can be fairly certain of an excellent vascular study of the mediastinum. With this technique, vascular pathology such as the SVC syndrome is easily diagnosed, and in most cases the underlying cause is determined.

References

Bechtold RE, Wolfman NT, Karstaedt N, Choplin RH. Superior vena cava obstruction: detection using CT. *Radiology* 1985; 157:485–487.

Kellman GM, Alpern MB, Sandler MA, Craig BM. Computed tomography of vena caval anomalies with embryologic correlation. *RadioGraphics* 1988; 8:533–556.

Moncada R, Cardella R, Demos TC, Churchill RJ, Cardoso M, Love L, Reynes CJ. Evaluation of superior vena cava syndrome by axial CT and CT phlebography. *AJR* 1984; 143:731–736.

Section 2

The Chest

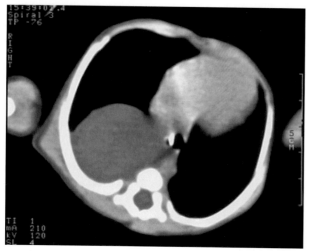

FIG. 29A. Non-contrast–enhanced CT

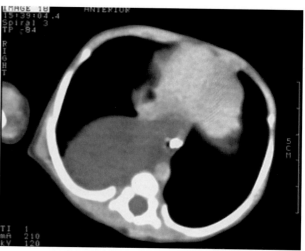

FIG. 29B. Non-contrast–enhanced CT

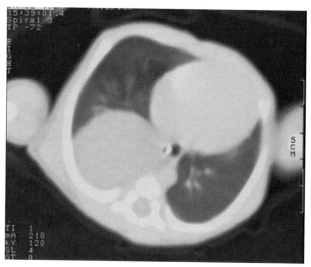

FIG. 29C. Non-contrast–enhanced CT

History

Newborn female noted to have an intrathoracic mass by ultrasound at 32 weeks gestation. Postnatally, chest ultrasound examination revealed an intrathoracic mass.

Findings

A spiral CT scan demonstrates a fairly homogeneous, low-density mass in the inferior portion of the right lower lung region. There is no evidence of any bronchi within the lesion. No associated bony abnormalities are seen. The lesion does not enhance significantly with contrast medium.

Diagnosis

Extralobar sequestration.

Discussion

Enhanced spiral CT scanning in this 1-day-old infant was successful without any sedation because of the ability to rapidly acquire image data and process it following completion of the examination. The study demonstrates a fairly homogeneous mass in the posterior portion of the right lower lung, without associated bony involvement or an air bronchogram. Multiplanar reconstructions showed the mass to be above the diaphragm. The differential diagnosis of a mass in this location in a newborn would include a neurogenic tumor as well as a cystic adenomatoid malformation and sequestration. The patient underwent surgery and the mass was found to be composed of immature lung tissue with marked lymphangiectasis and a systemic vascular supply consistent with extralobar sequestration.

There are classically two types of sequestration: interlobar and extralobar. Extralobar sequestration is more common in males, and up to 90% occur on the left side. There is also an association of extralobar sequestration with other congenital anomalies. Associated anomalies that may occur with extralobar sequestration include diaphragmatic defects.

Extralobar sequestrations have a separate pleural encasement that may be either above or below the diaphragm. In 77% of the 133 cases reviewed by Savic, extralobar sequestrations were found to lie between the lower lobe and the diaphragm.

In most cases, sequestrations are detected as a result of symptoms caused by pulmonary infection or as an incidental pulmonary mass on a chest radiograph. With the increased use of ultrasound, a growing number of cases are being discovered incidentally in utero. Spiral CT with narrow collimation and the rapid infusion of iodinated contrast medium should be able to fully define the lesion as well as reveal any anomalous systemic arterial supply.

References

Embryology of the lung and pulmonary abnormalities of developmental origin. In: Groskin SA (ed.): *Heitzman's The Lung: Radiologic-Pathologic Correlation*, St. Louis: CV Mosby, 1993.

Ikezoe J, Murayama S, Godwin JD, Done SL, Ver Schakelen JA. Bronchopulmonary sequestration: CT assessment. *Radiology* 1990; 176:375–379.

Savic B, Birtel FJ, Thalen W, Funke HD, Kroche R. Lung sequestration: report of 7 cases and review of 540 published cases. *Thorax* 1979; 34:96–101.

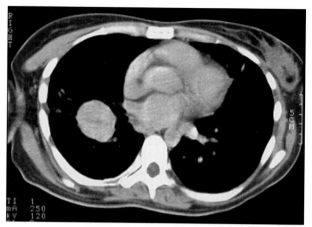

FIG. 30A. Non-contrast–enhanced CT

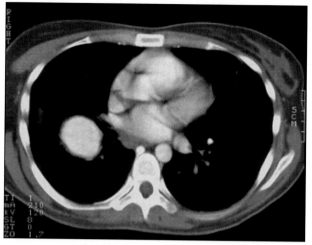

FIG. 30B. Contrast-enhanced CT

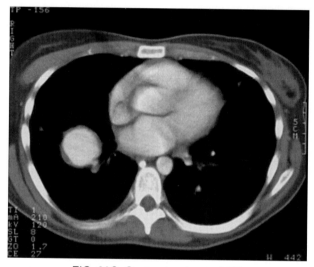

FIG. 30C. Contrast-enhanced CT

History

A 28-year-old female with a history of prior treatment for *Staphylococcus* endocarditis secondary to intravenous drug abuse. The patient was admitted with signs and symptoms of hepatitis. On routine admission chest x-ray, a mass was seen in the right hilum, which had appeared since prior radiographs.

Findings

A non-contrast-enhanced CT scan demonstrates a large right hilar mass. Spiral CT demonstrates marked enhancement of the mass, equal to that of the aorta. The mass appears to be in continuity with the right main pulmonary artery.

Diagnosis

Right pulmonary artery mycotic aneurysm due to *Staphylococcus* endocarditis.

Discussion

Spiral CT is especially useful in the evaluation of vascular pathology in the chest or abdomen. In the chest, several published studies have shown that a decreased volume of iodinated contrast medium may be used and successful studies performed for staging of lung cancer and the evaluation of aortic aneurysm or dissection. In the present case, a right hilar mass was seen whose etiology was uncertain. A primary vascular process or nodes were in the differential diagnosis. By using spiral CT and optimizing vascular enhancement, it was easy to define the process as a pulmonary artery aneurysm. The timing of data acquisition was approximately 50 seconds after initiation of injection of contrast material. In cases of suspected vascular pathology in the chest, an injection rate of 2 ml/sec for a total volume of 100 to 110 cc of contrast medium is satisfactory.

Pulmonary artery aneurysms are uncommon lesions. The causes are varied and include trauma, pulmonary hypertension, connective-tissue disease, and congenital processes. Mycotic pulmonary aneurysms are the result of an invasive infection of the arterial wall, and were once exceedingly rare but are becoming more common because of intravenous drug abuse. In a series reported by Navarro et al. of 68 mycotic pulmonary aneurysms, these lesions were the most common solitary lesions involving the pulmonary artery trunk or its major branches. Mycotic pulmonary aneurysms have also been described in patients who are intravenous drug abusers with endocarditis of a tricuspid pulmonic valve. A recent article by Loevner et al. noted that antemortem diagnosis is rare, with hemoptysis being a common terminal event. Currently, if pulmonary aneurysm is detected with spiral CT, then angiography may be performed with embolization. In the present case, the patient did develop hemoptysis and emergency resection of a pulmonary artery aneurysm with right lower lobe lobectomy was performed successfully.

Spiral CT should be used in the evaluation of any known or suspected mediastinal mass. The ability to synchronize the acquisition of data with contrast enhancement of major arterial and venous structures allows clear delineation of the presence of primary or secondary vascular processes.

References

Loevner LA, Andrews JC, Francis IR. Multiple mycotic pulmonary artery aneurysms: a complication of invasive mycormycosis. *AJR* 1992; 158:761–762.

Navarro C, Dickinson T, Kondlapoodi P, Hagstrom J. Mycotic aneurysms of the pulmonary arteries in intravenous drug addicts: report of three cases and review of the literature. *Am J Med* 1984; 76:1124–1131.

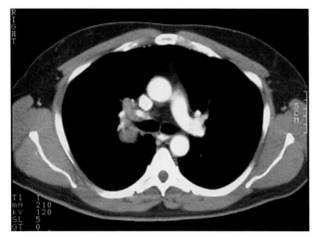

FIG. 31A. Contrast-enhanced CT

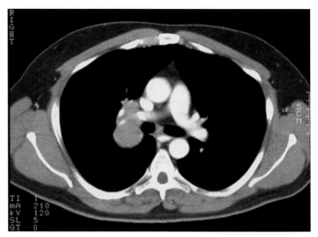

FIG. 31B. Contrast-enhanced CT

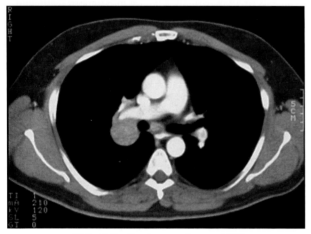

FIG. 31C. Contrast-enhanced CT

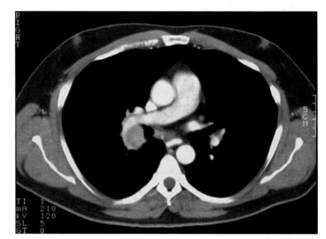

FIG. 31D. Contrast-enhanced CT

History

A 46-year-old male with a history of generalized weakness. Chest x-ray suggested the presence of a right hilar mass. A spiral CT scan was done to determine the extent of disease and its likely etiology.

Findings

A spiral CT scan of the chest demonstrates a large right hilar mass compressing the right pulmonary artery, though not apparently invading it. There is evidence of compression of the right main stem bronchus just past its origin, with no evidence of a postobstructive process. The differential diagnosis includes a primary lung cancer as well as lymphoma.

Metastatic disease to the mediastinum would also have to be a consideration. Inflammatory processes that involve the hilar region, such as tuberculosis or sarcoidosis, might also be considered, although sarcoidosis would be unlikely in light of the unilateral nature of the disease in this case.

Diagnosis

Hodgkin's disease.

Discussion

The present case shows the excellent mapping of the hilar regions provided by routine spiral CT with narrow collimation. This case uses 5 mm of collimation with reconstruction at 3-mm intervals. There is clear definition of the location of the pulmonary vessels and associated adenopathy. This study could be used as a guide for bronchoscopy and subsequent nodal biopsy.

Remy-Jardin et al. reviewed a series of spiral CT scans of the hilar region to try to determine the appearance of normal hilar lymph nodes and associated soft tissues on spiral CT. They then mapped the location of hilar lymph nodes and their relationships to the various segments of the pulmonary artery. They found that spiral CT accurately depicts normal hilar lymph nodes and their major anatomic relationships. The excellent mapping of the hilar regions by Remy-Jardin et al. is helpful both in defining the normal hilar regions and in carefully defining the anatomic landmarks in the region.

This case shows that the appearance of lymph nodes is often nonspecific, since the differential diagnosis in this case would be fairly extensive. Hodgkin's disease can present with hilar nodes as in the present case, and in this case the patient's constitutional symptoms suggested a malignancy.

Although routine dynamic CT can be used for evaluation of the hilar regions, it is somewhat difficult to maintain adequate contrast enhancement of the vessels throughout the study. This again is one of the advantages of spiral CT.

References

Remy-Jardin M, Duyck P, Remy J, et al. Hilar lymph nodes: identification with spiral CT and histologic correlation. *Radiology* 1995; 196:387–394.

Sone S, Higashihara T, Morimoto S, et al. CT anatomy of hilar lymphadenopathy. *AJR* 1983; 140:887–892.

Touliopoulos P, Costello P. Helical (spiral) CT of the thorax. *Radiol Clin North Am* 1995; 33:843–861.

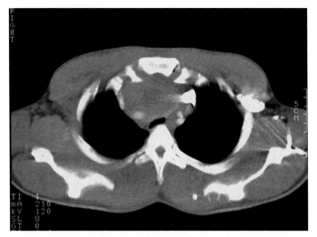

FIG. 32A. Contrast-enhanced CT

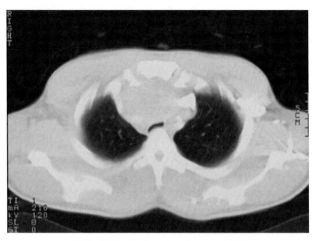

FIG. 32B. Contrast-enhanced CT

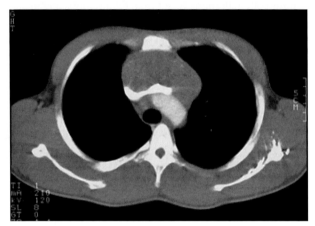

FIG. 32C. Contrast-enhanced CT

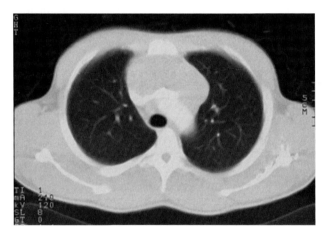

FIG. 32D. Contrast-enhanced CT

History

A 22-year-old male with increasing shortness of breath and dyspnea.

Findings

A spiral CT scan demonstrates a markedly narrowed upper airway, seen best on lung windows (Fig. 32B, D). On soft-tissue windows (Fig. 32A, C), a large tumor mass is seen encasing the mediastinum and involving the airway, causing the airway narrowing.

Diagnosis

Lymphoblastic lymphoma.

Discussion

The present case demonstrates a mass that is infiltrating the anterior mediastinum. The mass is of fairly homogeneous density, and in other scans extends upward into the neck. The airway is involved and is encased in a circumferential fashion by the tumor. The differential diagnosis is that of an anterior mediastinal mass, which in this age group tends to favor lymphoma, though other possibilities include teratoma and thymoma. The CT appearance of a homogeneous mass would tend to exclude teratoma, and the diffuse nature and airway involvement by the mass would tend to be extremely unusual for thymoma. This mass was biopsied and was indeed a lymphoma.

Lymphoma, despite its often bulky size, rarely involves the airway in our experience. In most cases, lymphoma displaces structures but does not invade them. In the present case, however, the trachea was encased and involved by tumor, causing the patient's clinical symptoms. The CT scan was used for planning radiation therapy, which was given immediately to prevent potential closure of the patient's airway.

In evaluating mediastinal masses, CT has nearly 100% accuracy in detecting lesions and localizing their origin. However, the differential diagnosis of lesions may also yield a conclusion if specific clinical findings are present, such as fat in a dermoid tumor or teratoma. However, in the case of a mass that tends to be infiltrating in the proper age group, lymphoma would be a most likely diagnosis.

References

Blank N, Castellino RA. The mediastinum in Hodgkin's and non-Hodgkin's lymphomas. *J Thorac Imag* 1987; 2:66–71.

Castellino RA, Blank N, Hoppe RT, Cho C. Hodgkin disease: contributions of chest CT in the initial staging evaluation. *Radiology* 1986; 160:603–605.

Sussman SK, Halvorsen RA Jr, Silverman PM, Saeed M. Paracardiac adenopathy: CT evaluation. *AJR* 1987; 149:29–34.

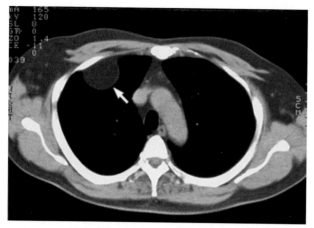

FIG. 33A. Contrast-enhanced CT

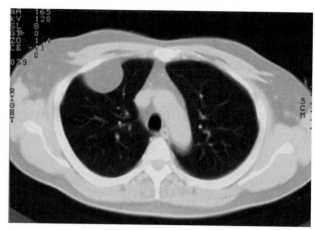

FIG. 33B. Contrast-enhanced CT

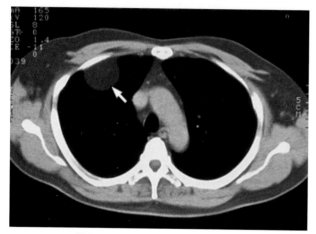

FIG. 33C. Contrast-enhanced CT

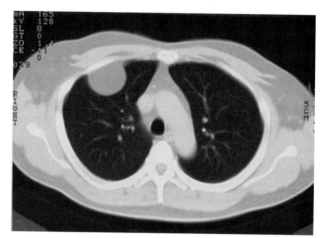

FIG. 33D. Contrast-enhanced CT

History

A 38-year-old male with a mass seen on chest x-ray. A CT scan was done for further evaluation.

Findings

A spiral CT scan demonstrates a pleural-based mass in the anterior portion of the right upper chest. The mass has a CT attenuation of around –100 Hounsfield units (HU) which is consistent with fat.

Diagnosis

Pleural lipoma.

Discussion

Spiral CT has been shown to provide accurate densitometry measurements, which can be used for the evaluation of parenchymal lung masses or renal masses. The use of spiral CT with narrow collimation and close interscan spacing allows the detection of fat or calcification even when it is subtle.

This case is somewhat unusual in that a lung mass was simulated by a pleural lipoma. CT clearly defines the location of the process and is able to exclude a parenchymal lesion. Because this is a benign process, no further investigation or workup was needed in this patient.

An article by Fisher and Godwin previously reported that normal thoracic fat on plain radiographs and CT scans can simulate a variety of disease processes. These include prominent chest-wall fat, which can simulate either pleural plaques or lung masses. Increased costal fat can be seen in association with adjacent lung thickening.

Similarly, increased fat can be seen in accessory fissures, along the phrenic nerve, or in other lung clefts. Other extrapleural fat collections that could be somewhat confusing include increased mediastinal fat, prominent cardiac fat pads, and retrosternal bands.

References

Fisher ER and Godwin JD. Extrapleural fat collections: pseudotumors and other confusing manifestations. *AJR* 1993; 161:47–52.

Glazer HS, Wick MR, Anderson DJ, et al. CT of fatty thoracic masses. *AJR* 1992; 159:1181–1187.

Proto AV. Conventional chest radiographs: anatomic understanding of newer observations. *Radiology* 1992; 183:593–603.

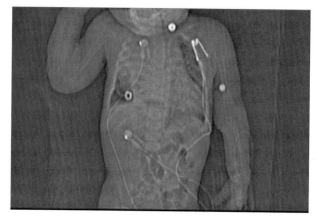

FIG. 34A. Scout

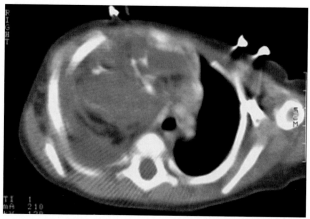

FIG. 34B. Contrast-enhanced CT

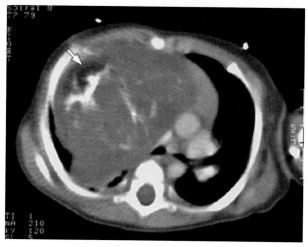

FIG. 34C. Contrast-enhanced CT

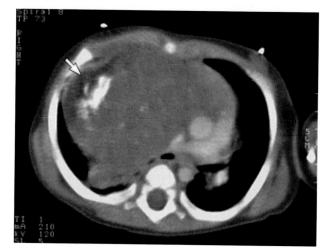

FIG. 34D. Contrast-enhanced CT

History

An 8-month-old female with symptoms of pneumonia. A spiral CT was done for evaluation of a mediastinal mass seen on a chest radiograph.

Findings

A spiral CT scan demonstrates a large anterior mediastinal mass that is eccentrically located to the right of the midline. The mass compresses the superior vena cava and displaces the heart to the left. There are areas of calcification and fat (arrow) within the tumor mass.

Diagnosis

Immature teratoma arising in the anterior mediastinum.

Discussion

Teratomas are neoplasms composed of tissue foreign to the site in which they occur, and typically represent two or more embryonic layers. Teratomas are typically slow growing, benign neoplasms of the anterior superior mediastinum that arise near or within the thymus gland. Posterior mediastinal teratomas are rare and represent less than 8% of all cases. In slightly more than half of cases, patients are symptomatic, partly because of a large tumor size and compression of mediastinal structures. Patients may present with cough, dyspnea, chest pain, or pulmonary infections. In younger patients, as in this case, large tumors may result in respiratory distress. There is also compression of the superior vena cava in this case, which has also been reported.

The CT scan in this patient demonstrates the classic findings of a teratoma, which include a mass with fat and calcification within it. Because of the increased sensitivity of CT for detection of fat and calcification, this diagnosis is typically an easy one. Fat–fluid levels may occur but were not present in the current case. As is typical of the calcifications in a teratoma, they may have a variety of appearances and may be focal, occurring within the cyst wall or capsule, or occur as dense sheets of tissue. Thick segmental areas of what appears to be calcification may in fact represent ossification within the tumor. This is similar to the findings in other teratomas, such as those in the ovary. The therapy in cases of teratoma is surgical excision of the mass, which provides a survival of nearly 100%.

The final pathologic diagnosis in this case was immature teratoma. In adults, immature teratomas may show aggressive behavior and may have a poor prognosis, while in children they typically have a good prognosis following resection.

References

Kenny JB, Carty HML. Infants presenting with respiratory distress due to anterior mediastinal teratomas: a report of three cases and a review of the literature. *Br J Radiol* 1988; 61:241–244.

Lewis BD, Hurt BD, Payne WS, et al. Benign teratomas of the mediastinum. *J Thorac Cardiovasc Surg* 1983; 86:727–731.

Rosado-de-Christenso ML, Templeton PA, Moran CA. Mediastinal germ cell tumors: radiologic and pathologic correlation. *RadioGraphics* 1992; 12:1013–1030.

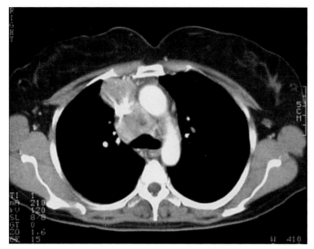

FIG. 35A. Contrast-enhanced CT

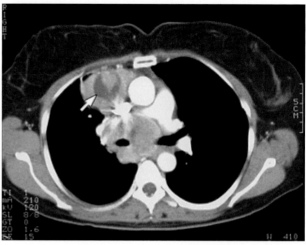

FIG. 35B. Contrast-enhanced CT

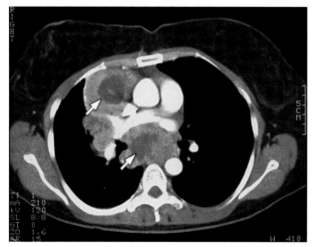

FIG. 35C. Contrast-enhanced CT

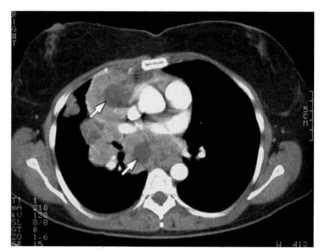

FIG. 35D. Contrast-enhanced CT

History

A 51-year-old female developed coldlike symptoms including a cough. The patient was initially treated with antibiotics, which did not totally relieve the symptoms. A chest x-ray revealed a mediastinal mass. A spiral CT scan was done for evaluation.

Findings

A spiral CT scan demonstrates extensive adenopathy in the anterior mediastinum, middle mediastinum, and posterior mediastinum. The tumor encases the right main pulmonary artery, with compression and narrowing, as well as compression of the superior vena cava. Interestingly, the nodes in the anterior and posterior mediastinum have areas of cystic change within them (arrows). One of the areas in the anterior mediastinum shows cystic change with what appears to be a mural nodule within it. In light of the patient's age and clinical history, the most favored diagnosis would be lymphoma. The second consideration would be metastatic disease to the mediastinum.

A fiberoptic bronchoscopy with biopsy was performed and demonstrated the tissue to be consistent with metastatic melanoma.

Diagnosis

Malignant melanoma involving the mediastinum.

Discussion

Malignant melanoma is a very aggressive neoplasm that can involve virtually every organ system. Malignant melanoma has a high propensity for extension to the lung. In one large autopsy series, lung metastases were found in 70% of patients. In fact, the thorax is the most common site of relapse in malignant melanoma, and this recurrence is often occult. Respiratory failure caused by replacement of lung tissue by tumor is the most common cause of death from malignant melanoma. It is uncommon, however, for the initial presentation, as in this case, to be in the chest. In most patients the melanoma is discovered as part of the staging workup or as a site of recurrence.

The true value of CT in the melanoma patient was established by Kostrubiak. In a series of 43 patients undergoing chest CT he found that there was a revision of the extent of disease based on CT scanning in 51.6% of the patients, and a change in therapy in 26%.

One of the CT findings we have noted in malignant melanoma is that the metastatic disease is often cystic, with a mural nodule. We have seen this appearance in the adrenal glands, spleen, kidney, and liver. In the present case, a similar finding was made, with the cystic zone in the mediastinum, containing a mural nodule within it.

Cystic changes in nodes are, however, not diagnostic for melanoma because they are also often seen in Hodgkin's disease, particularly in the form of Hodgkin's disease known as cystic Hodgkin's disease. Cystic changes may also be seen in patients with lymphoma following radiation therapy.

The role of spiral CT in the patient with melanoma is to help detect the full extent of disease. In the present case the value of rapid scanning is best defined by its demonstration of the encasement of the pulmonary artery by the tumor mass. In this study, involvement of the lung parenchyma and liver metastases were also noted. Spiral CT in this situation was able to scan both the chest and upper abdomen to provide an adequate staging of the patient in a single examination.

References

Fishman EK, Kuhlman JE, Schuchter LM, Miller JA III, Magid D. CT of malignant melanoma in the chest, abdomen, and musculoskeletal system. *RadioGraphics* 1990; 10:603–620.

Kostrubiak I, Whittle NO, Aisner J, et al. The use of computed body tomography in malignant melanoma. *JAMA* 1988; 259:2896–2897.

Patel JK, Didolkar MS, Pickren JW, Moore RM. Metastatic pattern of malignant melanoma. *Am J Surg* 1978; 135:807–810.

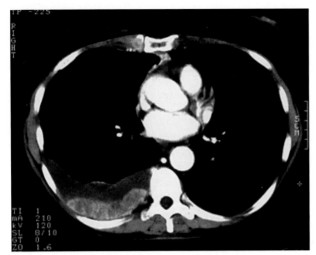

FIG. 36A. Contrast-enhanced CT

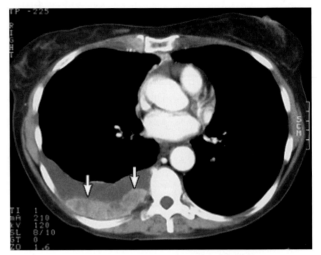

FIG. 36B. Contrast-enhanced CT

History

A 62-year-old female with a history of persistent cough and right shoulder pain. A chest x-ray demonstrated a mass in the right lung. A CT scan was done for further evaluation.

Findings

A spiral CT scan (Fig. 36A) demonstrates implants on the posterior right pleural surface (arrows). The implants are flat and run along the curvature of the chest wall. They are enhancing, and, therefore, distinct from the coexisting pleural effusion.

Diagnosis

Poorly differentiated adenocarcinoma of the right lung, with pleural implants.

Discussion

This case demonstrates the variable appearance of adenocarcinoma and the role of spiral CT in proper staging of this patient's disease. The CT scan suggests the diagnosis of a primary lung cancer, although the possibility of a mesothelioma or metastases to the pleura from an extrathoracic malignancy may be entertained.

Peripheral adenocarcinomas may grow directly into the pleura and simulate the appearance of a malignant mesothelioma. These tumor implants may enhance following bolus injection of contrast medium, which will better define their extent. The detection of chest-wall extension may be difficult unless actual bone destruction or muscle involvement is defined. Many cases may be indeterminate, and in these cases magnetic resonance imaging (MRI) may prove helpful if the patient has clinical symptoms. Involvement of the chest wall by lung cancer is an important finding in terms of determining the correct therapeutic approach. More aggressive management with local resection is now occurring in patients with chest-wall extensions of adenocarcinomas.

Neither CT nor MRI has been shown to be very accurate in determining chest-wall invasion from peripheral lung or pleural-based tumors. Although the accuracy varies in different series, reports have included standard CT as being inaccurate in 61% of cases. Although MRI is felt to be more accurate, no large series has documented its success as compared to CT. The role of spiral CT suggests that it may more helpful in determining the presence of tumor extension. Spiral CT provides thin sections and narrow interscan gaps, which make transition points easier to define. Also, use of multiplanar and sagittal reconstruction may prove very valuable in determining the true extent of tumors and helping to avoid the problem of partial averaging. However, this point will need to be defined with well-controlled series. Finally, spiral CT, by acquiring more sections of data per area of volume, provides a better opportunity for detecting even subtle involvement by showing the margins of consecutive sections. Although some papers have reported that spiral CT is more accurate than standard CT in the detection of lung nodules and involvement of the mediastinum, no one has yet documented it to be more accurate in the detection and definition of pleural disease.

The most accurate signs of chest-wall invasion on CT are rib destruction or extension beyond the pleural surface into the chest wall. This can be sometimes detected with spiral CT by enhancement of the soft tissues extending to the pleural space. Loss of normal extrapleural fat is suggestive of chest-wall invasion; however, this is not an absolute finding, and it may be more helpful on MRI than on CT.

References

Kuhlman JE, Bouchardy L, Fishman EK, Zerhouni EA. CT and MR evaluation of chest wall disorders. *RadioGraphics* 1994; 14:571–595.

Naidich DP. Helical computed tomography of the thorax—clinical applications. *Radiol Clin North Am* 1994; 32:759–774.

Rosado-de-Christenson ML, Templeton PA, Moran CA. Bronchogenic carcinoma: radiologic-pathologic correlation. *RadioGraphics* 1994; 14:429–446.

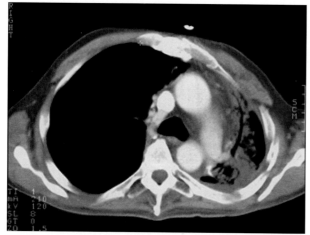

FIG. 37A. Contrast-enhanced CT

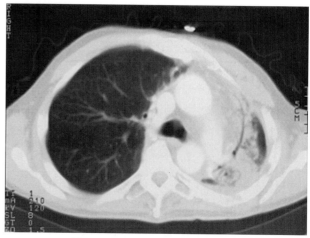

FIG. 37B. Contrast-enhanced CT

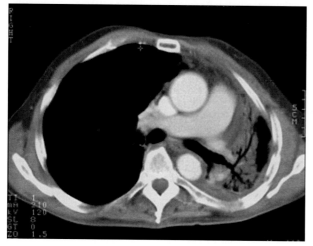

FIG. 37C. Contrast-enhanced CT

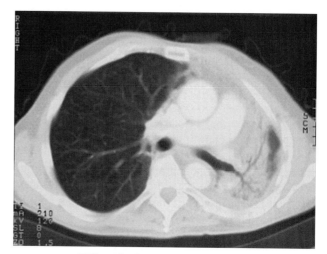

FIG. 37D. Contrast-enhanced CT

History

A 67-year-old male with a history of left lower lobe, non-small-cell lung cancer with prior left lower lung resection and postoperative radiation therapy.

Findings

A spiral CT scan demonstrates a loss of volume in the left hemithorax. Evidence of bronchiectasis is seen, with fibrosis of lung parenchyma also noted. No evidence of residual or recurrent tumor is seen.

Diagnosis

Radiation pneumonitis and fibrosis.

Discussion

One of the most important benefits of CT in the oncologic patient is its ability to distinguish changes caused by the patient's therapy from changes due to recurrent tumor. Radiation therapy alone or in combination with surgery is one of the more common procedures used for management of the patient with lung cancer. The changes caused by radiation therapy, and the potential pitfalls involved in evaluating a region that has had prior radiation therapy, are well known.

The role of spiral CT is to optimize enhancement of the vessels in the region of the mediastinum, and especially those in the hilar zones. This makes differentiation of areas of scarring, tumor recurrence, and vessel substantially easier. The present case is a good example of the ability of spiral CT to demonstrate the changes related to radiation and to show that there was no evidence of tumor recurrence.

The classic CT patterns in the lungs following radiation therapy have been addressed by Libshitz and Schuman, who divided these findings into four categories. The first category is a homogeneous, slightly increased attenuation of irradiated portions of the lung, typically at about 2 to 4 months after therapy. This represents the phase of classic radiation pneumonitis.

The second phase is that of patchy consolidation, which may simulate tumor recurrence with secondary infection. This typically occurs from 1 to 12 months after therapy.

The third pattern is a discrete consolidation conforming to radiation-therapy fields, and is typically one of the easiest patterns to recognize. This typically occurs at a minimum of 3 months after therapy, and represents the stage at which bronchiectasis is present.

The fourth and final phase is solid consolidation corresponding to therapy fields, with an associated loss of volume due to fibrosis, and represents an end-stage appearance. Bronchiectatic changes are invariably present at this time. This typically occurs 6 months after therapy. In most patients, radiation fibrosis will stabilize at 1 year after therapy. The present case corresponds to such an example, with extensive fibrosis and bronchiectatic changes. No tumor recurrence was noted.

References

Bluemke DA, Fishman EK, Kuhlman JE, Zinreich ES. Complications of radiation therapy: CT evaluation. *RadioGraphics* 1991;11:581–600.

Libshitz HL, Shuman LS. Radiation-induced pulmonary change: CT findings. *J Comput Assist Tomogr* 1984; 8:15–19.

Mah K, Poon PY, Van Dyk J, et al. Assessment of acute radiation-induced pulmonary changes using computed tomography. *J Compute Assist Tomogr* 1986;10:736–743.

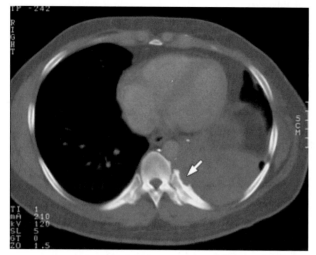

FIG. 38A. Contrast-enhanced CT

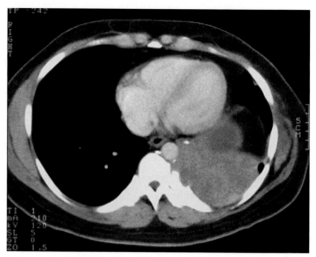

FIG. 38B. Contrast-enhanced CT

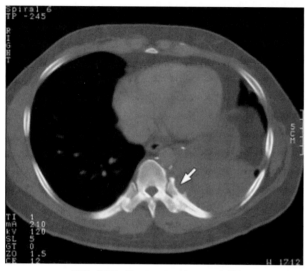

FIG. 38C. Contrast-enhanced CT

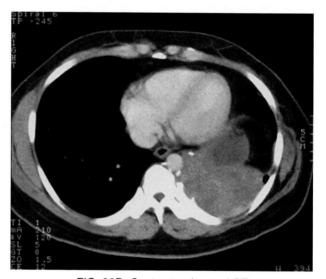

FIG. 38D. Contrast-enhanced CT

History

A 40-year-old male with a history of a left thoracotomy done 4 years earlier for resection of a spindle-cell sarcoma. A suspected recurrent tumor was seen on a routine radiograph prior to lumbar disc surgery.

Findings

A spiral CT scan demonstrates a soft-tissue mass that infiltrates the left lower lung with apparent bony involvement. The mass extends up to, but does not grow through, the diaphragm.

Diagnosis

Recurrent spindle-cell sarcoma of the chest.

Discussion

The lesion was biopsied and was consistent with recurrent disease from the primary tumor resected 4 years earlier. Spiral CT with narrow interscan spacing is the study of choice for evaluation of the lung parenchyma. It remains the dominant study for the detection of tumor recurrence in the oncology patient. In cases of disease near the diaphragm, it helps to localize disease extent and involvement.

Pulmonary sarcomas are rare, although two of the most common are leiomyosarcoma and fibrosarcoma (also referred to as spindle-cell sarcoma). These tumors can arise in the lung parenchyma, bronchial wall, or pulmonary artery. Intraparenchymal lesions usually occur in older patients and may present as smooth or lobulated masses. Extension into the chest wall may occur. It is often impossible to make a specific diagnosis without additional clinical information. Like all sarcomas, spindle-cell sarcomas are aggressive, and when located peripherally may invade the chest wall.

References

Guccion JG, Rosen SH. Bronchopulmonary leiomyosarcoma and fibrosarcoma: a study of 32 cases and review of the literature. *Cancer* 1972; 30:836.

Neoplastic Disease of the Lung. In: Groskin, SA (ed.): *Heitzman's The Lung: Radiologic-Pathologic Correlations.* St. Louis: CV Mosby, 1993, pp. 510–517.

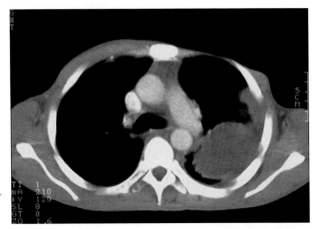

FIG. 39A. Contrast-enhanced CT

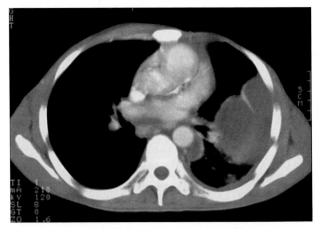

FIG. 39B. Contrast-enhanced CT

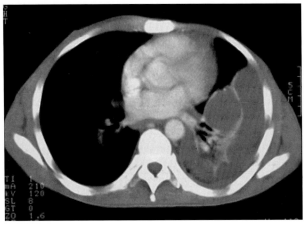

FIG. 39C. Contrast-enhanced CT

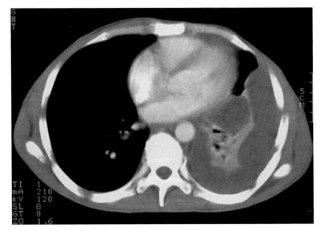

FIG. 39D. Contrast-enhanced CT

History

A 40-year-old male with a history of left-sided chest pain that was sharp and pleuritic in return. He also had a history of productive cough, fever, chills, and night sweats. The patient had a past medical history of recurrent squamous cell carcinoma of the neck, and had had a radical neck dissection done approximately 7 months earlier. The patient was human immunodeficiency virus (HIV) negative but did have a history of intravenous drug and alcohol abuse.

Findings

A spiral CT scan demonstrates a large homogeneous left pleural effusion that extends into the fissure and appears to be somewhat lobulated. Associated atelectasis is seen as well. There appears to be a relative loss of volume in the left hemithorax. No evidence of metastatic lung disease or adenopathy is seen.

Diagnosis

Empyema in the left chest secondary to *Staphylococcus aureus* infection.

Discussion

In the present case the clinical history suggests either a process related to metastatic disease or to infection. Spiral CT showed no evidence of metastatic head or neck tumor to the chest. Rather, there was an apparently loculated, multicompartmental left pleural effusion that had a mass effect resulting in atelectasis in the left lower lung. There was no evidence of pleural nodularity or extension or involvement of the chest wall. Spiral CT is helpful in distinguishing between pleural fluid and atelectasis, since atelectatic lung will commonly enhance. As in this, case, one may also see air bronchograms and vessels extending through atelectatic lung that are not seen within pleural fluid. The differential diagnosis in this case is centered around the cause of the pleural effusion, but in a patient with a history of intravenous drug abuse, fever, and other constitutional symptoms, one would be more suspicious of an empyema.

The patient did have a tap of pleural fluid that grew *Staphylococcus aureus*. Blood cultures subsequently were also positive. The patient was felt to have endocarditis resulting in the empyema. He was treated with antibiotics and had a chest tube inserted, which was eventually removed. He was discharged with antibiotic therapy.

CT has previously been shown to be an excellent modality for determining the presence and extent of pathology in the pleural space. Detection of pleural fluid and planning of therapy are two applications of CT scanning. In selected patients, pleural effusions may be loculated, particularly when infected, and it is important to make sure that adequate drainage is performed. In many cases, follow-up CT scans may be done, particularly if the patient is febrile, to exclude the possibility of an undrained collection. Although chest x-rays are very helpful in this regard, they may fail to clearly define the location and involvement of pleural fluid, especially in the face of concurrent atelectasis. Complications resulting in empyemas, including bronchopleural fistulas, can also be well seen with CT. Spiral CT would obviously have the advantage over routine CT in this application because thin sections can be obtained with a single breath-hold. Also, multiplanar reconstruction can prove helpful in these patients.

References

Baber CE, Hedlund LW, Oddson TA, Putman CE. Differentiating empyemas and peripheral pulmonary abscesses. *Radiology* 1980; 135:755–758.

Baldt MM, Bankier AA, Germann PS, Po;auschl GP, Skrbensky GT, Herold CJ. Complications after emergency tube thoracostomy: assessment with CT. *Radiology* 1995; 195:539–543.

Westcott JL, Volpe JP. Peripheral bronchopleural fistula: CT evaluation in 20 patients with pneumonia, empyema, or postoperative air leak. *Radiology* 1995; 196:171–181.

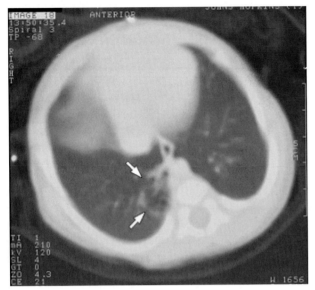
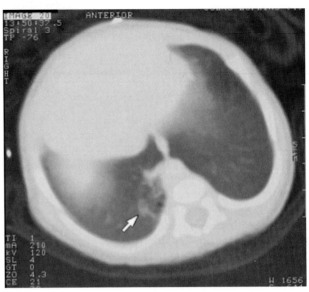

FIG. 40A. Contrast-enhanced CT   FIG. 40B. Contrast-enhanced CT

History

A newborn male delivered by spontaneous vaginal delivery at 39 weeks. A lung mass was seen on prenatal ultrasound examination.

Findings

Figures 40A and B are spiral CT scans obtained with 4 mm slice thickness and a reconstruction interval of 4 mm. The scans demonstrate a lesion in the posterior basilar segment of the right lower lung that is in part cystic, with tiny septations present within it (arrows). The lesion is not enhancing. Although the patient was not sedated, the images are of good quality with a 1-second spiral acquisition.

Diagnosis

Congenital cystic adenomatoid malformation.

Discussion

Cystic adenomatoid malformation (CAM) is an uncommon congenital lung lesion that represents approximately 25% of all congenital lung lesions. The vast majority of such lesions are found in the neonatal period, with up to 90% discovered during the first 2 years of life. CAM is slightly more common in males than females. Its clinical presentation typically include respiratory distress, cyanosis, or infection. In other cases, lesions may be discovered incidentally in utero on ultrasound examination. There are classically three types of CAM, with Type 1 being the most common. Type 1 is composed of one or more thin-walled cysts measuring 2 to 10 cm in diameter. They are accompanied by smaller cysts as well. In childhood, the CT appearance of CAM will depend on whether or not there is secondary infection present. In cases with infection, the classic thin-walled cysts are replaced by thicker walled cysts or even a mass-like presentation. As noted above, most cases are seen in early childhood, but a recent article reviewed a series of 7 patients who presented as adults between the ages of 21 and 61 years.

With the use of spiral CT, we are better able to examine the chest in patients who were classically unable to tolerate an examination because of the inability to remain still or to provide the necessary cooperation. The 1-day-old infant in the present case was scanned and the diagnosis made without the need for sedation. Spiral CT will play a major role in pediatric CT scanning.

In the differential diagnosis of this case of congenital CAM, one should also consider pulmonary sequestration, bronchogenic cyst, or prior infection with a pneumatocele appearance. Spiral CT with intravenous injection of contrast medium is helpful in distinguishing among these entities, as in the present case.

References

Panicek DM, Heitzman ER, Randall PA, et al. The continuum of pulmonary developmental anomalies. *RadioGraphics* 1987; 7:741–771.

Patz Jr EF, Müller NL, Swensen SJ, Dodd LG. Congenital cystic adenomatoid malformation in adults: CT findings. *J Comput Assist Tomogr* 1995; 19:361–364.

Rosado-de-Christenson ML, Stocker JT. Congenital cystic adenomatoid malformation. *RadioGraphics* 1991; 11:865–866.

Shackelford GD, Siegel MJ. CT appearance of cystic adenomatoid malformations. *J Comput Assist Tomogr* 1989; 13:612–616.

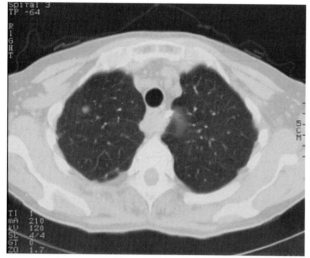

FIG. 41A. Non-contrast–enhanced CT

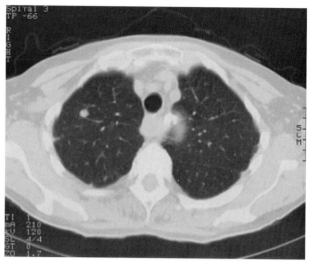

FIG. 41B. Non-contrast–enhanced CT

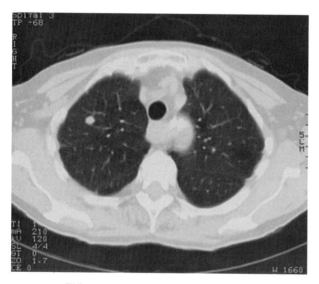

FIG. 41C. Non-contrast–enhanced CT

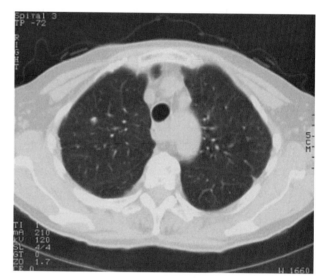

FIG. 41D. Non-contrast–enhanced CT

History

77-year-old female with a suspected nodule in the right upper lung on chest x-ray, as well as suspected mediastinal widening.

Findings

A sequential set of 4-mm-thick CT scans were reconstructed at 2-mm intervals. They clearly define the presence of a 7-mm right upper lung nodule. Note that the lesion is well seen in Figure 41B and 41C but can easily be missed in Figures 41A and D. The lesion is not calcified. The apparent mediastinal widening seen on chest radiography is an aberrant right subclavian artery, and not due to any associated adenopathy.

Diagnosis

Solitary pulmonary nodule (SPN) due to adenocarcinoma.

Discussion

One of the challenges of CT scanning is the detection and characterization of pulmonary nodules. Many of the earliest articles written about body CT defined its superiority in lesion detection to both plain chest radiographs and standard tomography. Several articles also demonstrated the superiority of CT for the detection of lesion calcification. Therefore, CT became the study of choice for evaluation of an SPN.

However, conventional CT also has potential limitations in lesion detection. Uneven levels of respiratory effort can result in missed lesions, a problem especially true in the lower lung fields. Spiral CT potentially solves this problem by acquiring all information during a single 24 to 32-second breath-hold.

Costello et al. reviewed a series of 20 patients with suspected pulmonary nodules less than 1 cm in size on plain chest radiographs. Conventional CT and 12-second spiral CT scans were done on these patients. Four nodules were detected with spiral CT that were missed on conventional CT. The mean size of the missed nodules was 4.5 mm. Buckley et al. reviewed a series of 67 spiral CT studies to determine whether the capability of increased data sampling with spiral CT could increase lesion detection. They found that by doubling the sampling interval from every 8 mm to every 4 mm, the detection rate increased by nearly 10% and the confidence level (as measured by false-positive studies) was also improved. In that study the increased data sampling yielded definite results for most lesions (482 vs. 431, $P < 0.025$) and fewer equivocal lesions (101 vs. 135, $P < 0.055$). The greatest effect was found in a reduced number of possible lesions (50 vs. 88, $P < 0.001$) and a reduced number of false-positive diagnoses made by less experienced radiologists.

References

Buckley JA, Scott WW Jr, Siegelman SS, Kuhlman JE, Urban BA, Bluemke DA, Fishman EK. Pulmonary nodules: effect of increased data sampling on detection with spiral CT and confidence in diagnosis. *Radiology* 1995; 196:395–400.

Costello P, Anderson W, Blume D. Pulmonary nodule: evaluation with spiral volumetric CT. *Radiology* 1991; 179:875–876.

Siegelman SS, Khouri NF, Leo FP, Fishman EK, Braverman RM, Zerhouni EA. Solitary pulmonary nodules: CT assessment. *Radiology* 1986; 160:307–312.

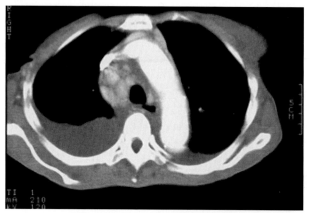

FIG. 42A. Contrast-enhanced CT

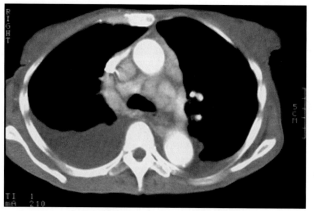

FIG. 42B. Contrast-enhanced CT

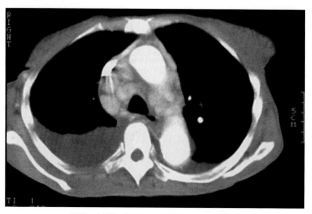

FIG. 42C. Contrast-enhanced CT

History

A 62-year-old female with a history of acute renal failure and mediastinal widening on chest radiography. The patient also had a history of congestive heart failure and reflux sympathetic dystrophy.

Findings

Spiral CT scan demonstrates extensive nodes in the pretracheal space and aortopulmonary window. The nodes are enhancing, but not the degree of the mediastinal structures. Bilateral pleural effusions are also present. The patient also has large subcarinal nodes.

Diagnosis

Castleman's disease of the mediastinum.

Discussion

A spiral CT scan of the chest demonstrates extensive mediastinal adenopathy. The nodes measured well over 1.5 cm in diameter. What is unique about the adenopathy is that the nodes are enhancing. The differential diagnosis of adenopathy in this location would include lymphoma, small-cell lung cancer, and metastatic disease to the mediastinum from primary tumors such as renal-cell carcinoma. Enhancement of the nodes would also suggest the possibility of an inflammatory etiology.

In most cases of adenopathy, the lymph nodes are of soft-tissue attenuation. In select cases, nodes have been known to cystic or necrotic. Cystic nodes are classically described in disease entities including testicular tumor and lymphoma. In other cases, lymph nodes are calcified, although this is typically due to granulomatous disease such as tuberculosis or histoplamosis. Calcified nodes may also be seen in pneumocystic infection. Occasionally, lymphoma will present with calcified nodes, although most cases of calcified nodes with lymphoma are usually secondary to prior radiation therapy. The presence of enhancing nodes is indeed very rare. We have seen several cases of enhancing nodes in metastatic melanoma, particularly when there is adenopathy in the axillary zone. Hypervascular nodes are typically associated with

Castleman's disease or angioimmunoblastic lymphadenopathy.

Castleman's disease is a benign condition intermediate on the spectrum between simple benign reactive lymph nodes and lymphoma. There are two main types described pathologically. The most common type has hyaline-type vascular nodes with proliferation of capillaries and follicles with associated hyalinization. Such patients are usually asymptomatic. Patients who are symptomatic usually have fever and weight loss, although cough, dyspnea, and hemoptysis may also be reported. The second type of Castleman's disease is termed the plasma-cell type and is less common, occurring in less than 20% of cases. In this type, plasma cells are found interspersed between normal and large lymphoid follicles. Plasma-cell-type disease is more commonly symptomatic and may involve a hypergammaglobulin anemia. The radiologic diagnosis of Castleman's disease is typically based on the presence of enhancing lymph nodes. For example, on a non-contrast-enhanced CT scan, it would be impossible to distinguish Castleman's disease from lymphoma. The mediastinum is the most common location of Castleman's disease, but it has also been described in the neck, retroperitoneum, axilla, and pelvis.

References

Castleman B, Iverson L, Menendex V. Localized mediastinal lymph-node hyperplasia resembling thymoma. *Cancer* 1956;9:822–830.

Feigin DS, Siegelman SS, Theros EG, King FM. Nonmalignant lymphoid disorders of the chest. *AJR* 1977; 129:221–228.

Ferreirós J, León Gómez N, Mata MI, Casanova R, Pedrosa CS, Cuevas A. Computed tomography in abdominal Castleman's disease. *J Comput Assist Tomogr* 1989;13:433–436.

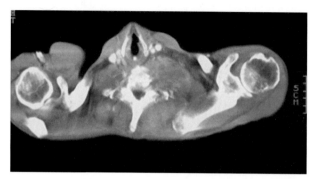

FIG. 43A. Contrast-enhanced CT

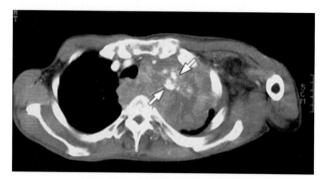

FIG. 43B. Contrast-enhanced CT

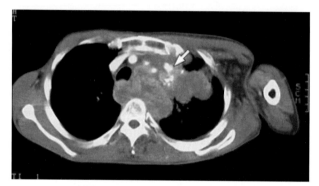

FIG. 43C. Contrast-enhanced CT

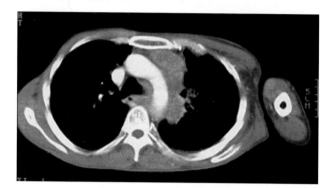

FIG. 43D. Contrast-enhanced CT

History

36-year-old male with a history of chest pain and fullness in the left cervical region.

Findings

A spiral CT scan demonstrates large necrotic lymph nodes in the left supraclavicular zone. Extensive tumor involves the anterior mediastinum, with areas of punctate calcification (arrows). The tumor also encases the aortic arch.

Diagnosis

Primary thymic carcinoma with neuroendocrine features.

Discussion

The spiral CT scan in this case demonstrates a very aggressive tumor that has grown through the chest wall into the lung apex, with destruction of the lower cervical spine and ribs. The mass is relatively avascular and has punctate calcification. The first diagnosis to be entertained would that of a very aggressive lung cancer such as a Pancoast tumor, with extension and destruction. It would be somewhat unusual for these tumors to have calcification as in the present case, but Pancoast tumor would still be the leading possibility. The second group of tumors would be those producing a primary anterior mediastinal mass; one possibility might be a lymphoma. Lymphoma can invade bone and can be fairly destructive. However, it is somewhat unusual for lymphoma to have calcifications unless the tumor has been irradiated. Other considerations in cases of aggressive tumors of the anterior mediastinum include sarcomas.

Thymic epithelial tumors represent approximately 15% of all mediastinal masses and can be classified as thymomas or thymic carcinomas. Thymomas tend to be more common, and although patients may present with clinical symptoms such as myasthenia gravis or red-cell aplasia, many cases are found incidentally in the older age population. Thymic carcinomas tend to be more aggressive than thymomas.

Thymic carcinomas represent a group of unusual epithelial neoplasms of the thymus characterized by a high degree of anaplasia. The tumors are more aggressive than invasive thymoma, with a poorer prognosis. Thymic carcinomas have nine variants based on cytologic characteristics, the most common being squamous and lymphoepithelioma like carcinomas. The average survival of patients with thymic carcinoma is less than 2 years. In a series of cases examined by Do et al., the tumors were solid anterior mediastinal masses with areas of necrosis. They were aggressive infiltrating tumors, and extension into the chest wall was not uncommon. Do et al. reviewed CT scans in patients with thymic carcinoma and found that in 92% there was invasion into the chest wall. Although direct extension by thymomas can occur, it is definitely more common in thymic carcinomas. Distant metastases were also much more common in the patients described by Do et al. Based on the CT appearance alone, it may be difficult to distinguish an invasive thymoma from a thymic carcinoma. Thymic carcinomas are not associated with myasthenia gravis, and more frequently involve mediastinal nodes and extrathymic metastases.

References

Do YS, Im JG, Lee BH, et al. CT findings in malignant tumors of thymic epithelium. *J Comput Assist Tomogr* 1995; 19:192–197.

Morgenthaler TI, Brown LR, Colby TV, Harper CM Jr, Coles DT. Thymoma. *Mayo Clin Proc* 1993; 68:1110–1123.

Rosado-de-Christenson ML, Galobardes J, Moran CA. From the Archives of the AFIP. Thymoma: radiologic-pathologic correlation. *RadioGraphics* 1992; 12:151–168.

Verstandig AG, Epstein DM, Miller WT Jr, Aronchik JA, Gefter WB, Miller T. Thymoma—report of 71 cases and a review. *Crit Rev Diagn Imag* 1992; 33:201–230.

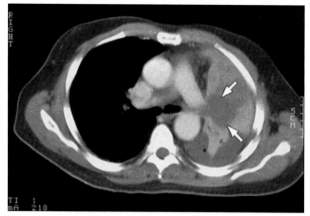

FIG. 44A. Contrast-enhanced CT

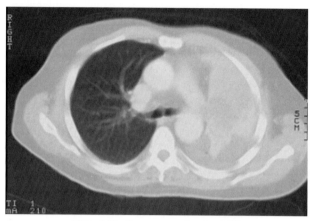

FIG. 44B. Contrast-enhanced CT

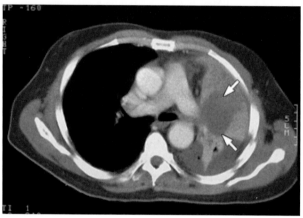

FIG. 44C. Contrast-enhanced CT

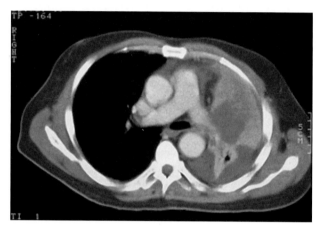

FIG. 44D. Contrast-enhanced CT

History

A 65-year-old male who presented with a 20-pound weight loss, dyspnea, and cough. A chest x-ray demonstrated opacification of the left hemithorax. A chest CT was done for further evaluation.

Findings

A spiral CT scan demonstrates total collapse of the left lung due to central tumor encasing the left main stem bronchus (arrows) just past its origin. There appear to be three different densities representing central tumor, postobstructive atelectasis, and pleural effusion.

Diagnosis

Squamous cell carcinoma of the lung.

Discussion

One of the most difficult diagnostic problems on chest CT has been outlining the precise location of central hilar tumors in the presence of distal atelectasis. This becomes of special importance when radiation therapy is planned and an attempt is made to limit the radiation field. Spiral CT, however, is useful in many of these cases. By acquiring data during maximum vascular enhancement, we can also take advantage of the fact that the atelectatic lung will enhance more than the central tumor, thereby providing a roadmap for the radiation therapist. Vessels extending through the atelectic lung may also be seen. Similarly, the ability to distinguish between tumor and atelectasis is helpful in determining sites for biopsy, whether percutaneously or bronchoscopic.

The frequency with which one can distinguish between tumor and atelectasis has not yet been described in any article in the literature. However, we appear to be seeing this more frequently. Properly timed scanning at 50 to 70 seconds after the initial administration of contrast material, appears to provide an ideal study.

One of the limitations of spiral CT is its inability to scan the entire lung with high resolution at a narrow collimation (1 to 2 mm). In the case of 2-mm collimation and a pitch of 2, a 32-second spiral will cover only 12.8 cm, about half of what is needed to scan an average-sized chest. In cases in which the entire lung needs to be scanned, a strategy is to combine a spiral CT of 5 to 8-mm sections at 4-mm increments with several high-resolution nonspiral CT scans at the end of the study. These scans may be obtained from the top of the aortic arch, moving caudally at 15 to 20-mm intervals. Another strategy might be to obtain back-to-back spiral scans, which will cover most of the chest. However, this may mean twice the radiation dose for a patient without a known malignancy (i.e., to evaluate suspected bronchiectasis).

References

Mayr B, Ingrisch H, Häussinger K, Huber RM, Sunder-Plassmann L. tumors of the bronchi: role of evaluation with CT. *Radiology* 1989; 172:647–652.

Primack SL, Lee KS, Logan PM, Miller RR, Müller NL. Bronchogenic carcinoma: utility of CT in the evaluation of patients with suspected lesions. *Radiology* 1994; 193:795–800.

Storto ML, Ciccotosto C, Patea RL, Spinazzi A, Bonomo L. Spiral CT of the mediastinum: Optimization of contrast medium use. *Eur J Radiol* 18(Suppl. 1)1994; S83–S87.

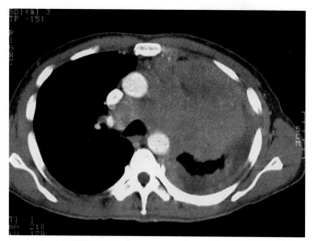

FIG. 45A. Contrast-enhanced CT

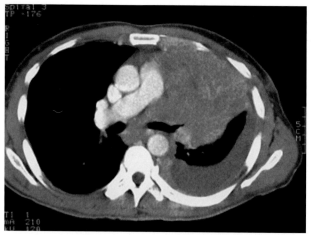

FIG. 45B. Contrast-enhanced CT

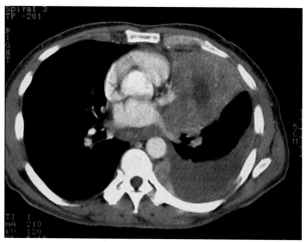

FIG. 45C. Contrast-enhanced CT

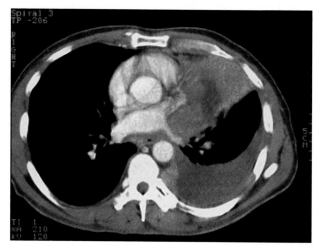

FIG. 45D. Contrast-enhanced CT

History

A 54-year-old male with a clinical presentation of cough, hemoptysis, and weight loss. The chest x-ray demonstrated near total opacification of the left hemithorax. A spiral CT scan was requested to define the extent of disease.

Findings

A spiral CT scan demonstrates a large tumor extending from the anterior mediastinum to the left hilar region, with encasement of the left main pulmonary artery. Invasion of the heart is also seen, with involvement of the left atrium. Pleural implants are also seen.

Diagnosis

Small-cell carcinoma of the lung.

Discussion

Several of the key advantages of spiral CT scanning in the staging of lung cancer are illustrated in this case. The involvement of the pleural surface with pleural implants is clearly defined. With spiral CT, pleural implants will enhance, but not to the degree of vessels. It is, however, easy to distinguish the pleural implants from underlying pleural fluid or atelectasis.

In terms of vascular encasement, coordination of contrast-medium injection with data acquisition allows for optimal opacification of vessels, which makes determination of encasement or invasion much easier. In this case, extension of tumor to involve the left atrium is a somewhat unusual finding, but is noted clearly. Small-cell carcinoma is often described as an infiltrating tumor, and this case is no exception to that.

Multiplanar reconstruction and/or three-dimensional imaging can be performed in this case, and can be used for planning therapy. Tumor volumetrics can also be obtained if clinically warranted.

References

Epstein DM, Stephenson LW, Gefter WB, et al. Value of CT in the preoperative assessment of lung cancer: a survey of thoracic surgeons. *Radiology* 1986; 161:423–427.

Glazer HS, Kaiser LR, Anderson DJ, et al. Indeterminate mediastinal invasion in bronchogenic carcinoma: CT evaluation. *Radiology* 1989; 173:37–42.

Quint LE, Francis IR, Wahl RL, Gross BH, Glazer GM. Preoperative staging of non-small cell carcinoma of the lung: imaging methods. *AJR* 1995; 164:1349–1359.

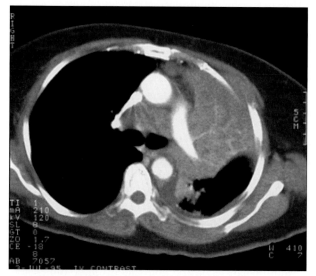

FIG. 46A. Contrast-enhanced CT

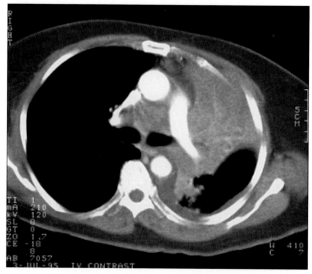

FIG. 46B. Contrast-enhanced CT

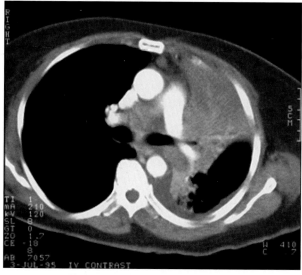

FIG. 46C. Contrast-enhanced CT

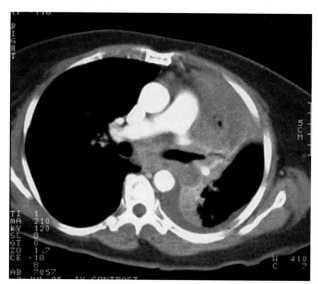

FIG. 46D. Contrast-enhanced CT

History

A 77-year-old female who came to the emergency room with complaints of worsening dyspnea and cough. A CT scan was ordered for further evaluation.

Findings

A spiral CT scan demonstrates encasement of the left pulmonary artery with vascular invasion. The patient has extensive tumor involving the left hilum, with encasement and vascular invasion of the left main pulmonary artery. There is also evidence of anterior mediastinal nodal involvement and pretracheal disease. Subtle air bronchograms are seen and postobstructive atelectasis is also noted.

Diagnosis

Encasement and invasion of the pulmonary artery by a poorly differentiated adenocarcinoma of the lung.

Discussion

The case clearly shows the compressed and invaded left pulmonary artery, with some subtle branching of vessels into the tumor in a neovascular-type pattern. We can also see air bronchograms present within the lesion. The extension of the tumor goes beyond the lung, through the intercostal space and into the chest wall, as seen in Figure 46C. Upon close inspection there is a differential attenuation between tumor, atelectatic lung, and pleural effusion, as best seen in Figure 46D. This demarcation is important if radiation therapy is planned.

CT has always played a major role in the detection, staging, and monitoring of therapy in lung cancer. The accuracy of CT has varied from one study to another, depending upon the criteria set and the population studied. One area of controversy has been the ability of CT to detect mediastinal invasion. Herman et al. reviewed a series of 90 patients with primary bronchogenic carcinoma who underwent CT with thoracic surgical staging and thoracotomy. They found CT to be insensitive in the detection of mediastinal invasion, although it had a high positive predictive value. The study used contiguous 1-cm-thick scans obtained after manual injection of contrast material. The author's results may be technique-limited, especially considering the representative figures in the paper, which show poor vascular enhancement. If these images are representative of the entire study population, one could postulate that the results would be better with spiral CT, power injection of contrast material, and closely spaced scans. The present case illustrates some of the advantages of spiral CT for these patients.

Although I can provide no specific accuracy data based on spiral CT data, this case shows the value of the spiral technique for detecting mediastinal invasion. In fact, an optimal technique might use 5-mm collimation, a 5-mm/sec table speed, and reconstructions at 3-mm intervals. In this case, multiplanar reformations could be done, which might have been helpful.

References

Gay SB, Black WC, Armstrong P, Daniel TM. Chest CT of unresectable lung cancer. *RadioGraphics* 1988; 8:735–748.

Herman SJ, Winton TL, Weisbrod GL, Towers MJ, Mentzer SJ. Mediastinal invasion by bronchogenic carcinoma: CT signs. *Radiology* 1994; 190:841–846.

Webb WR, Gatsonis C, Zerhouni EA, et al. CT and MR imaging in staging non-small cell bronchogenic carcinoma: report of the radiologic diagnostic oncology group. *Radiology* 1991; 178:705–771.

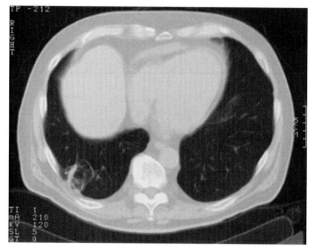

FIG. 47A. Axial CT

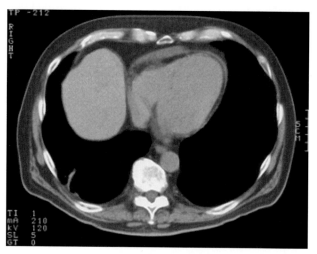

FIG. 47B. Axial CT

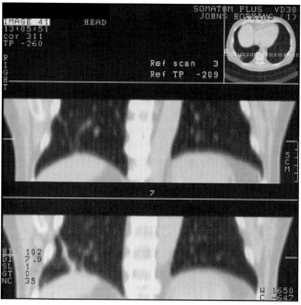

FIG. 47C. Coronal CT

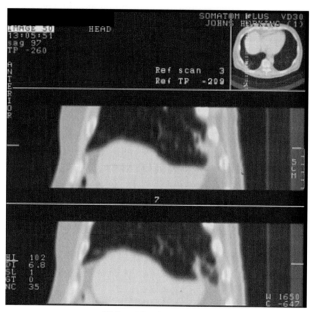

FIG. 47D. Sagittal CT

History

An 84-year-old male admitted to the hospital for resection of bladder cancer. A preoperative chest radiograph suggested a possible nodule in the right lower lung. A spiral CT was requested.

Findings

A spiral CT scan was done with 5-mm-thick sections, a table speed of 5 mm/sec, and data reconstructed at 3-mm intervals. On the transaxial views, the study demonstrates an area of linear scarring adjacent to an area of increased extrapleural fat. Coronal and sagittal reconstructions define the extent of the process from the diaphragm to the pleural surface.

Diagnosis

Inflammatory scar in the right lower lung.

Discussion

Spiral CT is the study of choice for evaluation of suspected parenchymal lung nodules, whether primary or metastatic. An article by Buckley et al. noted how an increase in the frequency of data sampling increased the accuracy of lesion detection. Similarly, an article by Collie et al. demonstrated that image acquisition with spiral CT is superior to that with conventional CT for assessment of pulmonary metastatic disease, based on a series of 23 patients and pulmonary phantoms.

One of the advantages of spiral CT is the ability to tailor the examination to the problem at hand. In the present case the key abnormality was suspected to be in the lower lung zone, next to the diaphragm. Since many of processes in the lower lungs arise from the diaphragm or pleural surface, it is important to obtain thin sections with narrow interscan spacing. This allows multiplanar reconstruction views to be obtained, which are often very helpful. Costello noted that multiplanar images generated from spiral CT data in the chest are generally free from the usual steplike artifacts, particularly if narrow collimation is used. Subsequently, he noted that coronal and sagittal reconstruction can be helpful in the evaluation of peridiaphragmatic masses, by depicting the underlying complex anatomic relationships. Although on the transaxial views in the present case it appears that the abnormality was due to an area of scarring or prior infection, multiplanar reconstructions made this more definitive by showing the linear nature of the process.

If multiplanar reconstruction is planned, the importance of narrow collimation and close interscan spacing cannot be overemphasized. Another point illustrated by this case is that in our daily practice we routinely scan patients from the apex down to the diaphragm. However, in patients in whom the suspected primary process is at the level of the diaphragm, or in patients who we feel cannot hold their breath for the duration of the spiral CT scan, we will scan in a caudal cranial direction, since the upper lung fields are less affected by minimal respiratory motion.

References

Buckley JA, Scott WW Jr, Siegelman SS, Kuhlman JE, Urban BA, Bluemke DA, Fishman EK. Pulmonary nodules: effect of increased data sampling on detection with spiral CT and confidence in diagnosis. *Radiology* 1995; 196:395–400.

Collie DA, Wright AR, Williams JR, Hashemi-Malayeri B, Stevenson AJM, Turnbull CM. Comparison of spiral-acquisition computed tomography and conventional computed tomography in the assessment of pulmonary metastatic disease. *Br J Radiol* 1994;67(797):436–444.

Costello P. Thoracic helical CT. *RadioGraphics* 1994; 14:913–918.

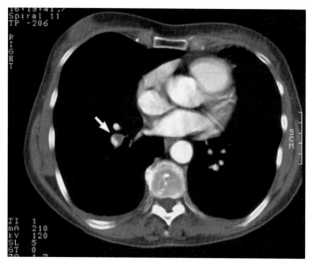

FIG. 49A. Contrast-enhanced CT

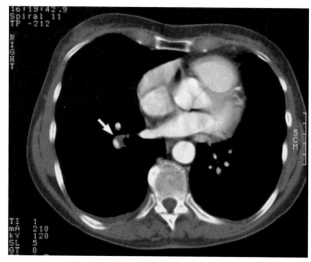

FIG. 49B. Contrast-enhanced CT

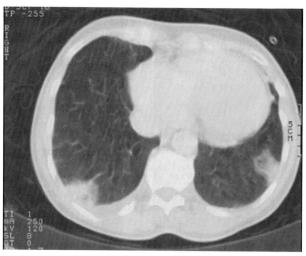

FIG. 49C. Contrast-enhanced CT

History

A 67-year-old female with severe pulmonary hypertension. The cause of the pulmonary hypertension was uncertain, but chronic pulmonary emboli was a clinical consideration.

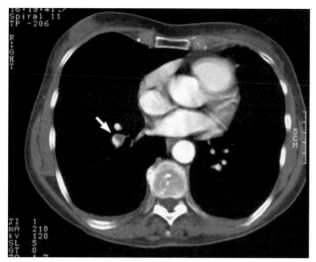

FIG. 49A. Contrast-enhanced CT

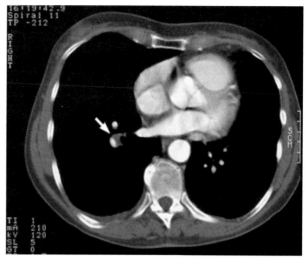

FIG. 49B. Contrast-enhanced CT

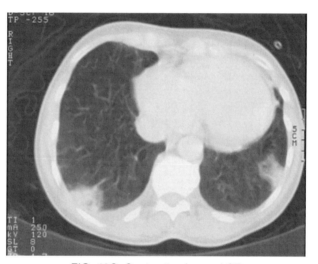

FIG. 49C. Contrast-enhanced CT

History

A 67-year-old female with severe pulmonary hypertension. The cause of the pulmonary hypertension was uncertain, but chronic pulmonary emboli was a clinical consideration.

Findings

A spiral CT scan demonstrates numerous small cavities in the lungs, as well as some dilated bronchi. There also appear to be small filling defects in the trachea, especially near the left main stem bronchus (arrow).

Diagnosis

Laryngotracheobronchial papillomatosis (LTP).

Discussion

The lung was biopsied, and the small mural nodules in the bronchial wall were found to be small papillomas with areas of focal atypia. No evidence of malignant change was seen.

LTP is a form of squamous-cell papilloma that most commonly occurs in the pediatric population. Although patients may not present until later in life, up to two-thirds of cases present by age 5. The tumor is usually caused by infection with the human papilloma virus (HPV), specifically HPV-II and HPV-6. Although most cases are confined to the larynx, the disease may occur more distally and into the lower respiratory tract. These cases are more difficult to treat, and recurrence is common. Malignant degeneration of a papilloma can occur.

Papillomas involving the lower airway are unusual. In an article by Kramer et al. they represented less than 1% of cases in 532 patients with LTP. When present, they are often multiple and may commonly cavitate. Air–fluid levels are not uncommon. These cavitary lesions have thin walls but may degenerate into squamous-cell carcinoma.

Spiral CT is helpful in these patients by defining the true extent of disease, and especially by defining smaller lesions. Complications like bronchial dilatation and bronchiectasis, as well as infection due to obstruction, can be well documented with spiral CT. Monitoring of these patients, including results following laser therapy, can be serially followed with spiral CT scanning.

References

Kramer SS, Wehunt WD, Stocker JT, Kashima H. Pulmonary manifestations of juvenile laryngotracheal papillomatosis. *AJR* 1985; 144:687–694.

McCarthy MJ, Rosado-de-Christenson ML. Tumors of the trachea. *J Thorac Imag* 1995; 10:180–189.

Takasugi JE, Godwin JD. The airway. *Semin Roentgenol* 1991; 26:175–190.

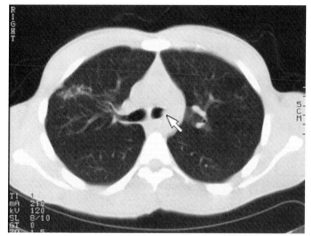

FIG. 48A. Non-contrast–enhanced CT

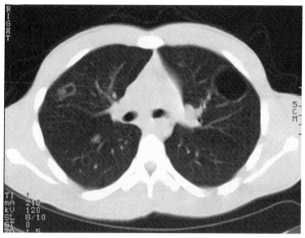

FIG. 48B. Non-contrast–enhanced CT

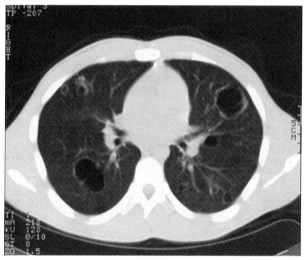

FIG. 48C. Non-contrast–enhanced CT

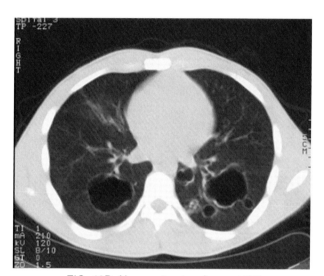

FIG. 48D. Non-contrast–enhanced CT

History

An 18-year-old male with a history of juvenile onset of bronchial papillomatosis. The study was done as a follow-up to an examination done 5 years earlier, to check for any progression of disease.

Findings

A spiral CT scan was done with 5-mm-thick sections, a table speed of 5 mm/sec, and data reconstructed at 3-mm intervals. On the transaxial views, the study demonstrates an area of linear scarring adjacent to an area of increased extrapleural fat. Coronal and sagittal reconstructions define the extent of the process from the diaphragm to the pleural surface.

Diagnosis

Inflammatory scar in the right lower lung.

Discussion

Spiral CT is the study of choice for evaluation of suspected parenchymal lung nodules, whether primary or metastatic. An article by Buckley et al. noted how an increase in the frequency of data sampling increased the accuracy of lesion detection. Similarly, an article by Collie et al. demonstrated that image acquisition with spiral CT is superior to that with conventional CT for assessment of pulmonary metastatic disease, based on a series of 23 patients and pulmonary phantoms.

One of the advantages of spiral CT is the ability to tailor the examination to the problem at hand. In the present case the key abnormality was suspected to be in the lower lung zone, next to the diaphragm. Since many of processes in the lower lungs arise from the diaphragm or pleural surface, it is important to obtain thin sections with narrow interscan spacing. This allows multiplanar reconstruction views to be obtained, which are often very helpful. Costello noted that multiplanar images generated from spiral CT data in the chest are generally free from the usual steplike artifacts, particularly if narrow collimation is used. Subsequently, he noted that coronal and sagittal reconstruction can be helpful in the evaluation of peridiaphragmatic masses, by depicting the underlying complex anatomic relationships. Although on the transaxial views in the present case it appears that the abnormality was due to an area of scarring or prior infection, multiplanar reconstructions made this more definitive by showing the linear nature of the process.

If multiplanar reconstruction is planned, the importance of narrow collimation and close interscan spacing cannot be overemphasized. Another point illustrated by this case is that in our daily practice we routinely scan patients from the apex down to the diaphragm. However, in patients in whom the suspected primary process is at the level of the diaphragm, or in patients who we feel cannot hold their breath for the duration of the spiral CT scan, we will scan in a caudal cranial direction, since the upper lung fields are less affected by minimal respiratory motion.

References

Buckley JA, Scott WW Jr, Siegelman SS, Kuhlman JE, Urban BA, Bluemke DA, Fishman EK. Pulmonary nodules: effect of increased data sampling on detection with spiral CT and confidence in diagnosis. *Radiology* 1995; 196:395–400.

Collie DA, Wright AR, Williams JR, Hashemi-Malayeri B, Stevenson AJM, Turnbull CM. Comparison of spiral-acquisition computed tomography and conventional computed tomography in the assessment of pulmonary metastatic disease. *Br J Radiol* 1994;67(797):436–444.

Costello P. Thoracic helical CT. *RadioGraphics* 1994; 14:913–918.

Findings

Spiral CT scans were obtained after infusion of 100 ml of Omnipaque 350, with an injection rate of 2.5 ml/sec. Figures 49A and B demonstrate a thrombus in the right pulmonary artery. Figure 49C demonstrates a wedge-shaped pleural-based process at the lung bases. The differential diagnosis of these processes as septic lesions or bland emboli will depend in great part on the clinical history.

Diagnosis

Pulmonary embolism.

Discussion

One of the most controversial and potentially important roles for spiral CT is in the evaluation of suspected pulmonary embolism. There have been several recent articles discussing the potential role of spiral CT in the evaluation of pulmonary embolism. The results reported in several of the initial articles were promising. Obviously the location and size of the pulmonary emboli will be critical in detecting their presence and the accuracy of CT in revealing them. Most authors state that in the first three branches of the pulmonary artery, embolism can be detected with spiral CT. A recent study by Goodman et al. tried to determine the sensitivity of helical CT as compared to pulmonary angiography in the detection of pulmonary embolism in patients with an unresolved clinical or scintigraphic diagnosis. Twenty patients were evaluated in the study, and 11 were ultimately proven to have pulmonary embolism. When the central vessels were analyzed, CT had a sensitivity of 86%, specificity of 92%, and likelihood ratio of 10.7. However, when subsegmental vessels were included, CT results dropped to 63%, 89%, and 5.7, respectively. Therefore, in the series, CT was 63% sensitive, with subsegmental emboli difficult to diagnose.

One criticism that can be made of the article by Goodman et al. is that 24-second spirals were used because of equipment limitations. Longer spiral sequences, which allow for better collimation, may be helpful. Also, faster spiral CT scans may be important. Many of the results that have been published have been achieved with the Imatron or Evolution scanner. The results with the Electron Beam scanner have been particularly promising, although its availability is somewhat limited.

In summary, then, spiral CT scanning may be a good technique for the evaluation of pulmonary embolism in an attempt to avoid angiography. When spiral CT is positive, the diagnosis is affirmative. The major question becomes what further studies, if any, are needed in the face of a negative CT scan. Further studies will help to determine what the correct imaging sequence should be.

References

Goodman LR, Curtin JJ, Mewissen MW, Foley WD, Lipchik RJ, Crain MR, Sagar KG, Collier BD. Detection of pulmonary embolism in patients with unresolved clinical and scintigraphic diagnosis: helical CT versus angiography. *AJR* 1995; 164:1369–1374.

Remy-Jardin M, Remy J, Wattinne L, Giraud F. Central pulmonary thromboembolism: diagnosis with spiral volumetric CT with the single-breath-hold technique — comparison with pulmonary angiography. *Radiology* 1992; 188:839–845.

Teigen CL, Maus TP, Sheedy PF II, Johnson CM, Stanson AW, Welch TJ. Pulmonary embolism: diagnosis with electron-beam CT. *Radiology* 1993; 188:839–845.

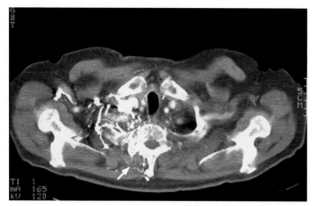

FIG. 50A. Contrast-enhanced CT

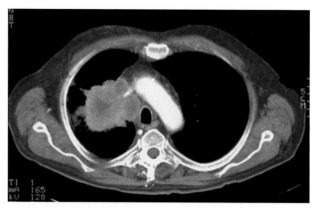

FIG. 50B. Contrast-enhanced CT

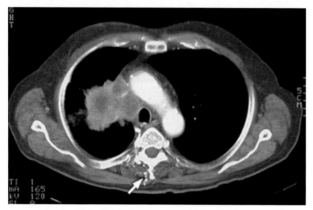

FIG. 50C. Contrast-enhanced CT

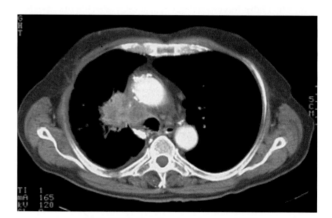

FIG. 50D. Contrast-enhanced CT

History

A 69-year-old male with a history of laryngeal carcinoma 5 years earlier. The patient had a recent weight loss and a chest x-ray showing mediastinal widening.

Findings

A spiral CT scan demonstrates extensive tumor extending from the right hilum into the pretracheal zone, with extension and near total occlusion of the superior vena cava. The azygos vein is dilated as a collateral vascular pathway. Collaterals are also seen along the right side of the spine (arrow).

Diagnosis

Small-cell carcinoma of the lung with extension into the mediastinum, and compression and near occlusion of the superior vena cava.

Discussion

The spiral CT in this case was used both for determining the extent of disease and for determining the best site for bronchoscopic biopsy. In terms of the staging of lung cancer, spiral CT should potentially help toward more accurate staging.

In the TNM staging classification, N_2 disease was previously defined as metastases to the mediastinal lymph nodes, and patients with such disease were felt not to be surgical candidates. Under the new classification system some cases of N_2 disease may be curable with resection of the primary tumor and mediastinal nodes, plus radiotherapy. The new classification also distinguishes between mediastinal nodal disease that is resectable (ipsilateral nodes and subcarinal nodes, as defined as N_2) and that which is not (contralateral mediastinal nodes plus ipsilateral and contralateral scalene and supraclavicular nodes), and which are designated N_3. This new division places an increasing burden on CT for correctly discriminating between these two populations in order to provide optimal patient management.

Spiral CT can provide this information with a tailored examination to both detect the presence of nodal disease and to accurately localize the nodes to the N classification. The classification is:

N0 = no demonstrable metastases or metastases to regional lymph nodes.

N1 = metastases to lymph nodes in the peribronchial or ipsilateral hilar region, or both, including direct extension.

N2 = metastases to ipsilateral mediastinal lymph nodes and subcarinal lymph nodes.

N3 = metastases to contralateral mediastinal lymph nodes, contralateral hilar lymph nodes, ipsilateral or contralateral scalene, or supraclavicular lymph nodes.

The key role for spiral CT is to detect and define nodal location. Thin collimation with narrow interscan spacing, as well as multiplanar reformatting, may prove very successful in this application.

References

Naidich DP. Helical computed tomography of the thorax: clinical applications. *Radiol Clin North Am* 1994; 32:759–774.

Stitik FP. The new staging of lung cancer. *Radiol Clin North Am* 1994; 32:635–647.

Watanabe Y, Shimizu J, Oda M, et al. Aggressive surgical intervention in N2 non-small cell cancer of the lung. *Ann Thorac Surg* 1991; 51:253–261.

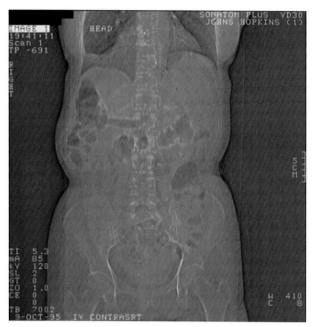

FIG. 51A. Scout

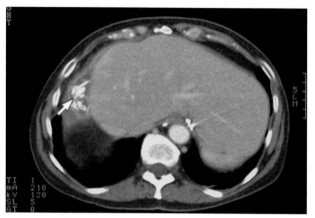

FIG. 51B. Axial contrast-enhanced CT

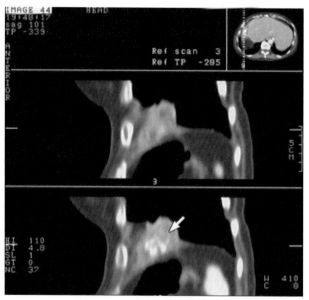

FIG. 51C. Sagittal contrast-enhanced CT

History

A 55-year-old female had a hepatic resection for hepatoma approximately 25 years earlier. The patient did well over the intervening years, although she most recently developed repeated episodes of right lower lung pneumonia. A plain radiograph suggested a foreign body at the level of the right hemidiaphragm, although it was unclear whether or not it was above or below the diaphragm.

Findings

CT with multiplanar reconstruction and three-dimensional imaging defined the suspected foreign matter as a retained surgical sponge (arrow) located above the hemidiaphragm.

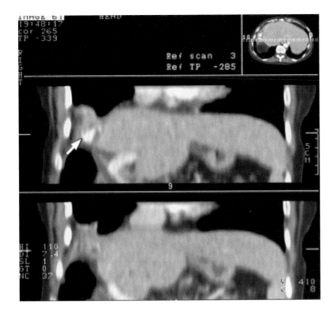

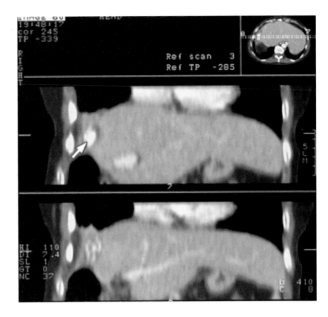

FIG. 51D. Coronal contrast-enhanced CT

FIG. 51E. Coronal contrast-enhanced CT

Diagnosis

Retained surgical sponge from surgery approximately 25 years earlier.

Discussion

Retained surgical sponges and towels (gossypibomas) are uncommon complications of surgery, owing in part to careful attention at the time of surgery to sponge and towel counts. However, there is occasionally human error and a sponge, towel, or surgical instrument may be inadvertently left inside the patient.

In select cases the error is located early in the postoperative period through findings on routine postoperative films or from complications such as postoperative abscess or bowel obstruction. In other cases the foreign matter may not be detected for years after surgery.

One of the important differential diagnostic points in these cases is to recognize the retained surgical sponge or towel and not confuse it with a primary or recurrent tumor. Several articles over the past few years have described the CT findings in cases of retained sponges or towels, which include a cys-

tic mass, a mass with air bubbles simulating an abscess, or a mass simulating matted bowel loops.

The present case is interesting both from the perspective of the delay in diagnosis and also for the problem of defining the location of the object. The patient's primary disease process was intraabdominal, and it was thought that the foreign matter should be below the diaphragm. However, the spiral CT multiplanar and three-dimensional images showed it to be above the diaphragm. This allowed the surgeon to plan the site of excision to remove the foreign matter, which was apparently contributing to the patient's clinical symptoms. Spiral CT is especially useful for peridiaphragmatic processes, through combining thin-section CT with narrow interscan spacing to yield high-quality reformatted images, which are not usually possible with routine dynamic CT scanning.

References

Buy JN, Hubert C, Ghossain MA, Malbec L, Bethoux JP, Ecoiffier JC. Computed tomography of retained abdominal sponges and towels. *Gastrointest Radiol* 1989; 14:41–45.

Caprio F, Lanza R, Amoroso L, Cerioni M, Carotti L. CT findings of surgically retained sponges and towels (gossypibomas). *Eur Radiol* 1993; 3:383–385.

Choi BI, Kim SH, Yu ES, Chung HS, Han MC, Kim CW. Retained surgical sponge: Diagnosis with CT and sonography. *AJR* 1988; 150:1047–1050.

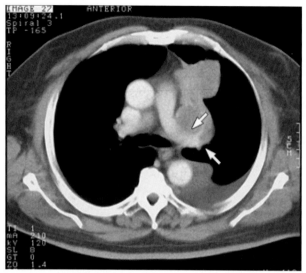

FIG. 52A. Contrast-enhanced CT

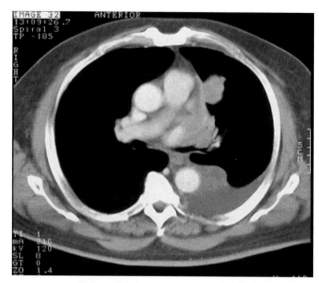

FIG. 52B. Contrast-enhanced CT

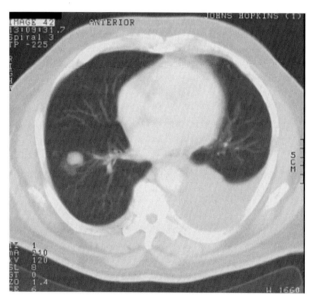

FIG. 52C. Contrast-enhanced CT

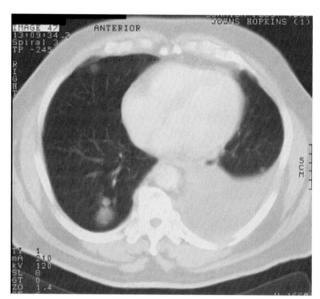

FIG. 52D. Contrast-enhanced CT

History

A 68-year-old male with a history of large-cell lymphoma diagnosed 2 years earlier. The tumor was localized to the abdomen and chemotherapy and radiation therapy was used. The patient did well until a recent development of cough and chest pain.

Findings

A spiral CT scan demonstrates tumor encasing the left hilum and pulmonary artery (arrows). A left pleural effusion and implants are seen. Multiple right lung nodules are also noted.

Diagnosis

Recurrent non-Hodgkin lymphoma of the lung, mediastinum, and pleural space.

Discussion

CT is currently the study of choice for the detection, staging, and follow-up of the patient with lymphoma. CT is ideal for this group of patients because of the potential of the disease process to involve multiple different organs and organ systems, with a wide range of appearances. CT can quantitate disease, including the generation of tumor volumes and the measurement and quantitation of absolute response.

In the chest, CT most often is used to detect mediastinal, hilar, or axillary adenopathy. However, involvement of the lung parenchyma is not uncommon, especially as a site of relapse of disease. In these cases, care must be taken to distinguish recurrent tumor from other processes such as infection (pneumonia) or radiation injury.

The most common CT appearance of parenchymal disease is a mass or masslike consolidation larger than 1 cm. The second most common finding is a nodule less than 1 cm in size. Other findings include alveolar or interstitial infiltrates, pleural-based masses or effusions, and peribronchial or perivascular thickening with or without atelectasis.

Spiral CT is well suited for the evaluation of these patients, in providing a volume of information with user-selected parameter sampling. Accurate and detailed information about the lung, mediastinum, and pleura is provided in a single examination.

References

Castellino RA. Hodgkin disease: practical concepts for the diagnostic radiologist. *Radiology* 1986; 159:305–310.

Khoury MB, Godwin JD, Halvorsen R, Hanun Y, Putman CE. Role of chest CT in non-Hodgkin lymphoma. *Radiology* 1986; 158:659–662.

Lewis ER, Caskey CI, Fishman EK. Lymphoma of the lung: CT findings in 31 patients. *AJR* 1991; 156:711–714.

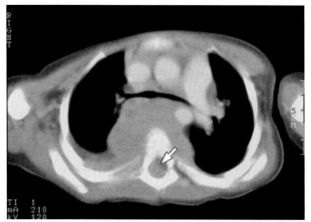

FIG. 53A. Non-contrast–enhanced CT

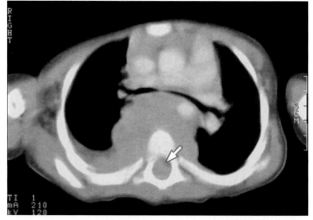

FIG. 53B. Non-contrast–enhanced CT

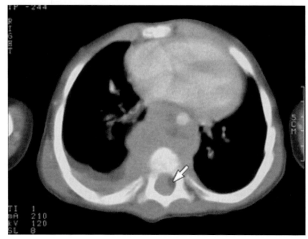

FIG. 53C. Non-contrast–enhanced CT

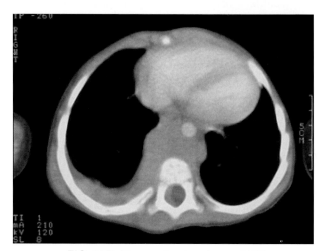

FIG. 53D. Non-contrast–enhanced CT

History

A 2½-year-old child presented with abdominal pain. Subsequent work-up demonstrated a Stage IV neuroblastoma. A spiral CT scan of the chest was obtained for evaluation, based on mediastinal widening seen on plain radiographs.

Findings

A spiral CT scan demonstrates a large posterior mediastinal mass that encases the aorta and lifts it off the spine. The left atrium is displaced forward as well. There is extension of tumor into the spinal canal, with displacement and compression of the spinal cord (arrows).

Diagnosis

Neuroblastoma involving the posterior mediastinum, with intraspinal extension.

Discussion

The posterior mediastinum is involved by a wide range of masses, the most common being of vascular or neurogenic origin. The posterior mediastinum can also be involved by inflammatory processes, whether they arise within the spine or extend to this region. In addition, pathology related to the aorta, including aneurysms or congenital vascular abnormalities, can cause apparent mediastinal widening due to posterior mediastinal masses.

Most neuroblastomas arise in the adrenal gland, but can extend throughout the abdomen as well as up into the chest. In the present case the patient's clinical presentation was due to the adrenal neuroblastoma, but there was involvement of the posterior mediastinum as well. In approximately 14% of cases of neuroblastoma the lesion is primarily intrathoracic.

Neurogenic tumors are commonly paravertebral, with intraspinal extension often occurring. Enlargement of the neural foramina or pressure erosion of the adjacent rib is not uncommon. In the present case, spiral CT allowed a successful study to be performed with adequate enhancement, which helps define the compression of the left atrium and encasement of the aorta. Spiral CT also provided the ability to see an enhancing tumor mass within the spinal canal and a clear fat plane between the extension of neuroblastoma and the spinal cord. Spiral CT also provides the opportunity for multiplanar reconstruction. In cases of neuroblastoma with intraspinal extension, multiplanar reconstruction can define the full extent of involvement. In these cases the multiplanar reconstruction may serve as a template for planning of radiation therapy.

In this 2½-year-old child, the differential diagnosis of the posterior mediastinal mass as presented in this case would also include lymphoma, although direct extension into the spinal canal would be uncommon.

References

David R, Lamki N, Fan S, et al. The many faces of neuroblastoma. *RadioGraphics* 1980; 9:859–882.

Kawashima A, Fishman EK, Kuhlman JE, Nixon MS. CT of posterior mediastinal masses. *RadioGraphics* 1991; 11:1045–1067.

Kumar AJ, Kuhajda FP, Martinez CR, Fishman EK, Jezic DV, Siegelman SS. Computed tomography of extracranial nerve sheath tumors with pathological correlation. *J Comput Assist Tomogr* 1983; 7:857–865.

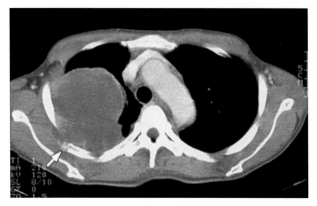

FIG. 54A. Contrast-enhanced CT

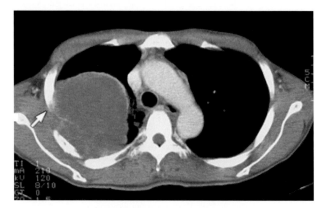

FIG. 54B. Contrast-enhanced CT

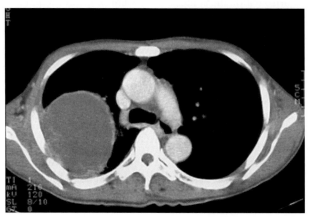

FIG. 54C. Contrast-enhanced CT

History

A 42-year-old male with a history of human immunodeficiency virus (HIV) infection and a CD4 cell count of approximately 90 mm³. The patient had a history of anaplastic lung cancer and presented with right-sided chest pain. The study was done to evaluate the extent of disease and to determine the cause of the patient's chest pain.

Findings

Spiral CT scan demonstrates a 9-cm mass with extension into the pleural surface and chest wall, with subtle rib erosion. A mass was also present in the contralateral lung.

Diagnosis

Anaplastic carcinoma of the lung with invasion of the pleura and right chest wall.

Discussion

One of the difficulties in the accurate staging of lung cancer occurs with peripheral lung masses extending to the pleural surface. Multiple articles have been written in the past noting that CT is less than optimal for determining chest-wall invasion in lung cancer unless definite extension through the chest wall is noted. In many of these cases, magnetic resonance imaging (MRI) has been suggested as a potential study that might better determine extension by showing changes in signal intensity within the chest wall. Also, select images in nonaxial planes (including the coronal, sagittal, and oblique planes) could be helpful in determining extension. Spiral CT provides many of the same capabilities as MRI. The present case, although not a subtle one, definitely defines the extension into the chest wall. One can clearly see that on the enhanced scan that there is enhancement of the mass involving the pleural surface, and associated rib destruction.

In an article by Kuriyama et al., spiral CT scans were obtained in 42 consecutive patients with peripheral bronchogenic carcinoma. Conventional two-dimensional and three-dimensional reconstructions of imaged data were reviewed by three observers, who reached a decision by consensus. Of the 42 patients, 12 had visceral pleural invasion, 5 had parietal invasion, and 25 had no evidence of pleural invasion. The visceral pleural invasion was identified on transaxial CT in two patients and on three dimensional reconstruction in 11 patients. Parietal pleural invasion was identified on transaxial CT in two patients and by three-dimensional reconstruction in 3 patients. The authors concluded that three-dimensional reconstruction supplementing transaxial images is valuable in the assessment of pleural invasion by peripheral bronchogenic carcinoma. One note is that Kuriyama et al. did not use multiplanar reconstruction, which can prove very valuable. Another potential problem with the study was that the three-dimensional reconstructions used were shaded-surface displays. Shaded-surface display may be inaccurate at interfaces, and could potentially result in false-positive or false-negative studies. It has been our experience that the use of multiplanar reconstruction, particularly in the coronal mode, may be very helpful in determining chest-wall involvement. Finally, the ability of spiral CT to provide closer interscan spacing on a routine basis may also prove very helpful in determining chest-wall invasion in cases in which it may only be seen on select images.

References

Fortier M, Mayo JR, Swensen SJ, et al. MR imaging of chest wall lesions. *RadioGraphics* 1994; 14:597–606.

Jafri SZH, Roberts JL, Bree RL, Tabor HD. Computed tomography of chest wall masses. *RadioGraphics* 1989; 9(1):51–68.

Kuriyama K, Tateishi R, Kumatani T, et al. Pleural invasion by peripheral bronchogenic carcinoma: assessment with three-dimensional helical CT. *Radiology* 1994; 191:365–369.

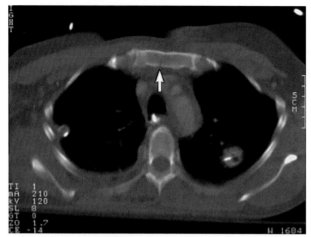

FIG. 55A. Contrast-enhanced CT

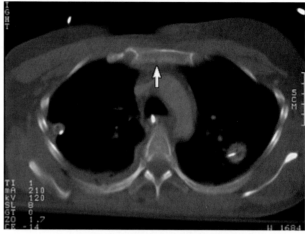

FIG. 55B. Contrast-enhanced CT

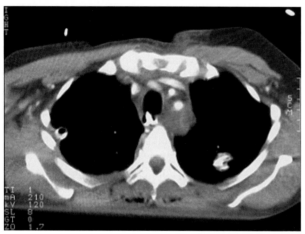

FIG. 55C. Contrast-enhanced CT

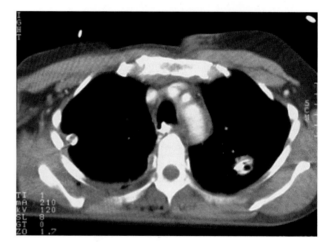

FIG. 55D. Contrast-enhanced CT

History

A 27-year-old female with a steering-wheel injury following a high-speed vehicular accident. Chest tubes were inserted because of pneumothoraces, and multiple rib fractures were noted. A spiral CT scan was done to rule out traumatic aortic dissection.

Findings

Spiral CT scan demonstrates a subtle fracture through the sternum (arrow). Contrast-enhanced image acquisition demonstrates evidence of mediastinal hematoma but no evidence of dissecting aneurysm.

Diagnosis

Mediastinal hematoma and sternal fracture following a motor-vehicle accident.

Discussion

Spiral CT has been shown to have a wide range of vascular applications. Its role in the evaluation of traumatic aortic injury is a topic of recent interest. A detailed analysis of the topic was recently presented by Gavant et al. These authors reviewed 1,518 patients with nontrivial trauma to the chest who had helical CT. Of these patients, 127 had abnormal CT scans of the mediastinum or aorta and underwent thoracic aortography. Twenty-one aortic injuries were identified that ranged from intimal flaps to complete aortic disruption. The authors found that helical CT was more sensitive than aortography (100% vs. 94.4%) but less specific (81.7% vs. 96.3%) in the detection of aortic injuries in patients who underwent both examinations. The authors concluded that spiral CT of the chest was in fact effective in screening critically injured patients with possible blunt thoracic aortic injuries.

Gavant et al. went as far as to list potential guidelines for radiologic evaluation of the aorta. They felt that if medical triage to aortography is based on the detection of mediastinal hematoma, no further evaluation of the thoracic aorta is necessary if spiral CT shows no abnormality involving the aorta or mediastinum. If there is a mediastinal hematoma but the aorta is normal, then no further evaluation is necessary. If there is a mediastinal hematoma but findings involving the aorta are indeterminate or inadequate to exclude injury, then aortography should be performed. An editorial by Trerotola enthusiastically found favor with the article by Gavant et al., but did note that a multicenter trial is probably needed before spiral CT can be defined as the single modality for evaluating thoracic injuries. Potential problems include injury to vessels off the aortic arch, which may not be seen on spiral CT.

The importance of spiral CT is emphasized by a recent article by Hunink and Bos, who did a cost–effect analysis of using CT for trauma. In this analysis, based on routine dynamic CT, the authors found that triage by CT is highly cost-effective if several guidelines are used.

References

Gavant ML, Menke PG, Fabian T, Flick PA, Graney MJ, Gold RE. Blunt traumatic aortic rupture: detection with helical CT of the chest. *Radiology* 1995; 197:125–133.

Hunink MGM, Bos JJ. Triage of patients to angiography for detection of aortic rupture after blunt chest trauma: cost-effectiveness analysis of using CT. *AJR* 1995; 165:27–36.

Trerotola SO. Can helical CT replace aortography in thoracic trauma? *Radiology* 1995; 197:13–15.

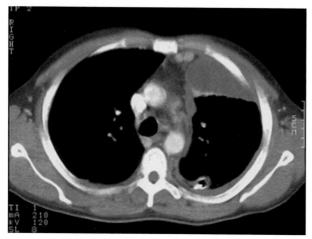

FIG. 56A. Contrast-enhanced CT

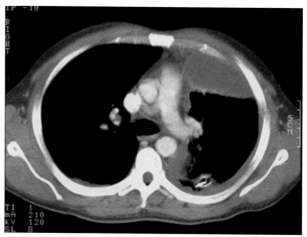

FIG. 56B. Contrast-enhanced CT

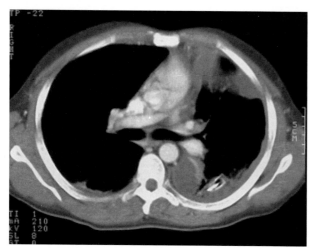

FIG. 56C. Contrast-enhanced CT

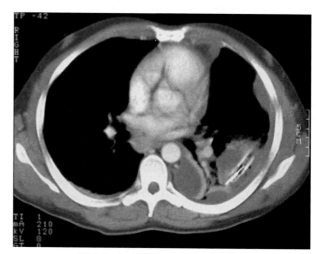

FIG. 56D. Contrast-enhanced CT

History

A 36-year-old male with a history of fever, productive cough, and pleuritic chest pain. A chest x-ray demonstrated a right pleural effusion and a chest tube was inserted. Despite the chest tube the patient had persistent fever. A CT study was requested for further evaluation.

Findings

A spiral CT scan demonstrates a loculated anterior left pleural effusion. The posterior left pleural effusion has a chest tube within it, but there is still a focal collection near the paraspinal region that is not drained. Small anterior mediastinal nodes are also seen. The patient was referred to thoracic surgery for evaluation.

Diagnosis

Undrained empyema of the left lung.

Discussion

Because of the patient's persistent fever and the spiral CT findings, a left lateral thoracotomy with rib resection and chest-tube placement was done, with evacuation of an empyema of the left chest. Culture of the fluid revealed growth of *Klebsiella* and heavy growth of *Enterobacter aerogenes*. The patient was treated with antibiotics and chest-tube drainage. The empyematous process resolved and he was discharged 2 weeks later.

This case is an excellent example of the usefulness of CT scanning in general, and of spiral CT specifically for the evaluation of pleural processes. In the present case the patient did have a pleural effusion but it had been thought to have been adequately drained until the patient did not respond to broad-spectrum antibiotics and chest-tube placement. In this case the chest x-ray showed a persistent infiltrate but no definite effusion, and a spiral CT scan was requested for further evaluation.

The spiral CT demonstrated that there were at least two collections that were not being satisfactorily drained. In the left lower lung, an area of atelectasis is seen just posterior to the left pulmonary artery and between the atelectatic lung and the spine. Although a lower chest tube is in place, this focal collection, which may be walled off, was not drained. There is also a large collection in the anterior portion of the left chest. However, no evidence of complication, such as extension through the chest wall or underlying lung abscess, was seen. Several articles in the radiologic literature have discussed the role of CT scanning in the evaluation and characterization of pleural pathology. Himmelman and Callen found a significant correlation between pleural-fluid loculations and pleural-fluid chemistries. In addition, they found that in 7 of 9 empyemas and 10 of 20 exudates the collections could be described on CT as loculated. In 30% of cases, pleural-fluid loculation was identified only by CT or sonography. None of these findings was noted in a patient with transudate effusion.

Spiral CT does enhance all of the classic signs used to help distinguish between a pleural effusion and parenchymal disease process. In addition, spiral CT can be used for monitoring the response to therapy and for complications of chest-tube placement including placement within the fissure or lung, as well as collections that are inadequately drained by a misplaced chest-tube. In select cases, spiral CT can also be used to help guide chest-tube placement into particularly difficult collections.

References

Baber CE, Hedlund LW, Oddson TA, Putman CE. Differentiating empyemas and peripheral pulmonary abscesses. *Radiology* 1980; 135:755–758.

Himmelman RB, Callen PW. The prognostic value of loculations in parapneumonic pleural effusions. *Chest* 1986; 90:852–856.

Westcott JL, Volpe JP. Peripheral bronchopleural fistula: CT evaluation in 20 patients with pneumonia, empyema, or postoperative air leak. *Radiology* 1995; 196:175–181.

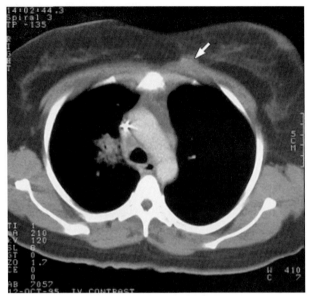

FIG. 57A. Contrast-enhanced CT

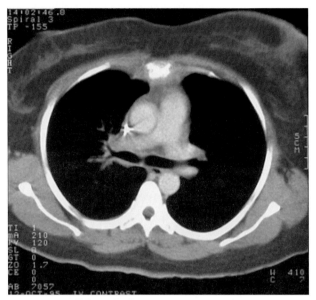

FIG. 57B. Contrast-enhanced CT

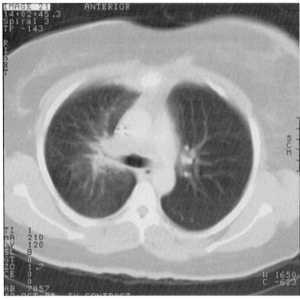

FIG. 57C. Contrast-enhanced CT

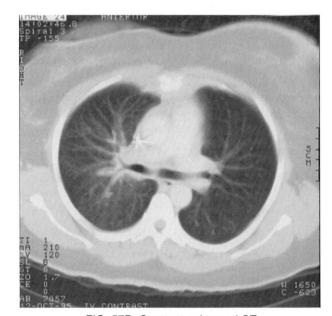

FIG. 57D. Contrast-enhanced CT

History

A 39-year-old female with a history of breast cancer. The patient had increasing shortness of breath. The study was done for further evaluation of extent of disease.

116

Findings

A Spiral CT scan demonstrates evidence of tumor in the anterior mediastinum, with involvement of the internal mammary nodes and left pectoralis major muscle (arrow). Skin thickening of the left breast is also seen. Evidence of involvement of the sternum is noted. On lung windows, evidence of tumor spread is seen in a pattern with increased nodularity around the vessels.

Diagnosis

Breast cancer with lymphangitic spread into the right lung and spread into the mediastinum and chest wall.

Discussion

The present case shows a typical pattern of spread of breast cancer. There is involvement of the mediastinal nodes with infiltration of the internal mammary region as well as involvement of the pectoralis muscle. There is evidence of spread into the lung parenchyma, with a classic pattern of lymphangitic spread. The patterns of lymphangitic spread seen on high-resolution CT have been described in several key articles. Müller described some of the classic high-resolution CT findings in lymphangitic spread of carcinoma, which included smooth or nodular peribronchial interstitial thickening, smooth or nodular interlobular septal thickening, prominence of lobular coarse structures, and smooth or nodular thickening of the fissures.

The findings of lymphangitic spread are especially well documented when comparing the right and left lung parenchyma. What is well illustrated by this case is that spiral CT should be used in both the evaluation of the mediastinum and the lung parenchyma. This was successfully done in a patient who was noticeably short of breath.

In regard to the value of spiral CT versus conventional CT for evaluation of the lung parenchyma, Paranjpe and Bergin found that CT scans of the lung obtained with the spiral and conventional modes at collimations at 5 and 8 mm showed no difference in resolution. However, spiral CT would be somewhat less optimal at collimations of 1 and 3 mm. The authors found that spiral CT with a bone-display algorithm provided the best solution, and that this had more effect on image quality than table speed or a linear interpolation algorithm.

Our experience has been very similar, and we have not documented any cases in which a spiral CT missed interstitial disease noted on routine dynamic scanning. In patients with interstitial spread of lung disease, the patient's shortness of breath often makes routine dynamic CT difficult. Although at first pass one might think that it would be impossible for these patients to hold their breath satisfactorily, we have not found this to be the case. For patients who feel that they would be unable to hold their breath for the proper period of time, we have found that shallow breathing works extremely well.

References

"Diseases characterized primarily by reticulonodular or nodular opacities." In: Webb WR, Mu;auller NL, Naidich DP (eds.): High resolution CT of the lung. New York: Raven Press, 1992, pp. 71–87.

Paranjpe DV, Bergin CJ. Spiral CT of the lungs: optimal technique and resolution compared with conventional CT. *AJR* 1994; 162:561–567.

Stein MG, Mayo J, Mu;auller NL, Aberle DR, Webb WR, Gamsu G. Pulmonary lymphangitic spread of carcinoma. *Radiology* 1987; 162:371–375.

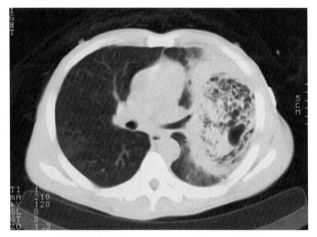

FIG. 58A. Non-contrast–enhanced CT

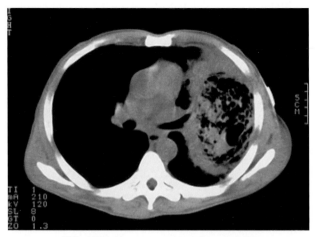

FIG. 58B. Non-contrast–enhanced CT

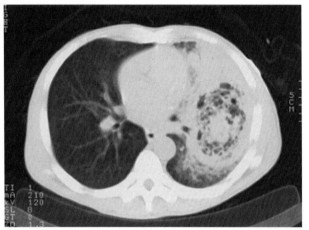

FIG. 58C. Non-contrast–enhanced CT

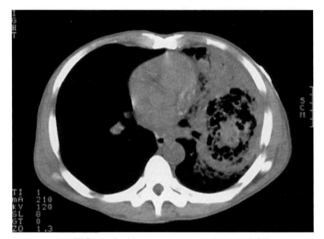

FIG. 58D. Non-contrast–enhanced CT

History

A 57-year-old male with a long history of cigarette smoking and alcohol abuse. He was admitted with a history of hemoptysis and a productive cough. A spiral CT scan was requested to rule out a central lung mass.

Findings

A spiral CT scan demonstrates a necrotizing infiltrate in the left lung, without a central obstructing process. Destruction of lung parenchyma is noted.

The patient died the next morning, and an autopsy was performed that revealed a necrotizing pneumonia with gangrene, involving both the left upper and lower lobes. The patient died from massive hemorrhage due to erosion of small pulmonary vessels by the necrotizing pneumonia.

This case of pulmonary gangrene is unusual and represents a process in which marked lung necrosis develops with occlusion of small arteries and veins. The necrotic lung sloughs from the visceral pleura and may collect in a central cavity. *Klebsiella* is the most common organism in such cases, although it they also result from *pneumococcus* infection. In the current case, the destruction of the lung parenchyma is very clear, with multiple cystic spaces.

CT is especially good for evaluation of the lung parenchyma and defining the extent of disease. In patients who are short of breath, as in this case, spiral CT can be used for successful completion of the examination.

Diagnosis

Necrotizing pneumonia with pulmonary gangrene and hemorrhage.

References

O'Reilly GV, Dee PM, Otteni GV. Gangrene of the lung: successful medical management of three patients. *Radiology* 1978; 126:575–579.

"Pneumonia and lung abscess." In: Groskin, SA (ed.): *Heitzman's The Lung: Radiologic-Pathologic Correlations.* St. Louis: CV Mosby, 1993, pp. 196–198.

The Gall Bladder
and
Bile Ducts

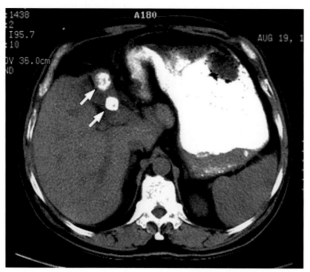

FIG. 59A. Non-contrast–enhanced CT

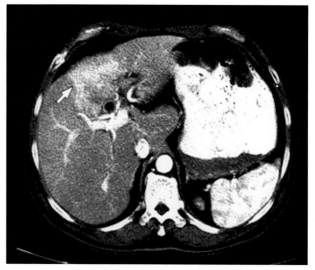

FIG. 59B. CT:arterial phase

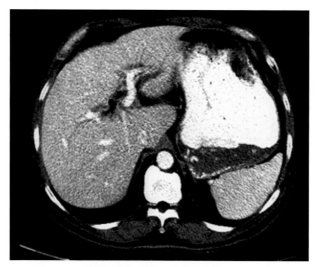

FIG. 59C. CT:venous phase

History

Acute cholecystitis. Rule out liver abscess.

Findings

Figure 59A is a non-contrast-enhanced CT scan of the liver demonstrating multiple calcified gallstones (arrow). In Figure 1B, which is an arterial-phase image of a biphasic spiral CT examination, note the focal area of increased enhancement within the medial segment of the left hepatic lobe (arrow). The focal area demonstrates straight margins along its periphery. Figure 59C is a scan obtained during the portal-venous phase, demonstrating normal hepatic enhancement in this area.

Diagnosis

Transient increased hepatic attenuation adjacent to the gallbladder in acute cholecystitis.

Discussion

This patient with acute cholecystitis demonstrates a focal area of increased attenuation adjacent to the gallbladder fossa during arterial-phase images. Yamashita et al. reported a similar finding in five patients with proven acute cholecystitis. The location of the focal area of enhancement was typically the medial segment of the left lobe of the liver. A characteristic pattern of enhancement was noted, with straight margins along the periphery of the area of enhancement. This pattern is different from most tumors, which are typically rounded.

It is hypothesized that the focal area of increased attenuation is related to localized hyperemia in association with early venous drainage adjacent to the inflamed gallbladder. It is also possible that there may be anomalous venous return in this area, and that the segment is largely perfused by hepatic arterial flow. This observation is much more apparent during early spiral CT scanning of the liver, particularly during the arterial phase of a biphasic study.

References

Yamashita K., Jin M.J., Hirose Y., et al. CT finding of transient focal increased attenuation of the liver adjacent to the gallbladder in acute cholecystitis. *AJR* 1995; 164:343–346.

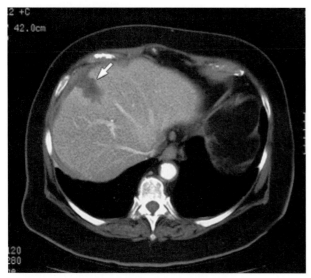

FIG. 60A. Contrast-enhanced CT

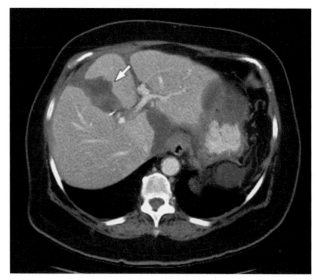

FIG. 60B. Contrast-enhanced CT

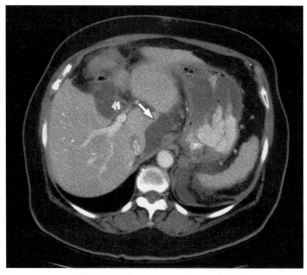

FIG. 60C. Contrast-enhanced CT

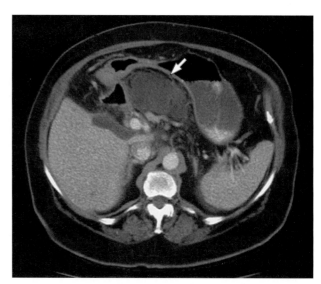

FIG. 60D. Contrast-enhanced CT

History

Persistent right upper quadrant pain following laparoscopic cholecystectomy.

Findings

Figure 60A–C are contrast-enhanced spiral CTs of the liver. Note in Figure 60A and B a laceration of the right lobe of the liver in close proximity to the main interlobar fissure between the right and left lobes (arrow). Notice in Figure 60C and D low-density fluid in both the superior recess (Figure 60C, arrow) and main portion of the lesser sac (Figure 60D, arrow). The water-density fluid is consistent with bile.

Diagnosis

Hepatic laceration and bile leak following laparoscopic cholecystectomy.

Discussion

Spiral CT is an excellent method to diagnose complications of laparoscopic cholecystectomy. The most common complications include bile leak, abscess, hemorrhage, and hepatic laceration. This patient did not have ongoing hemorrhage, and so the small hepatic laceration was treated conservatively. However, because of a persistent bile leak, an endoscopically placed common bile duct stent was inserted. At endoscopic retrograde cholangiopancreatography (ERCP) there was evidence of extravasation of contrast material from the region of the cystic duct, suggesting that the cystic duct was inadequately ligated during surgery. The patient made an uneventful recovery following biliary stenting. The stent was removed 3 months later.

References

Cervantes J, Roja GA, Ponte R. Intrahepatic subcapsular biloma. A rare complication of laparoscopic cholecystectomy. *Surg Endosc* 1994; 8:208–210.

Moran J, Del Grosso E, Wills JS, Hagy JA, Baker R. Laparoscopic cholecystectomy: imaging of complications and normal postoperative CT appearance. *Abdom Imag* 1994; 19:143–146.

Walker AT, Brooks DC, Tumeh SS, Braver JM. Bile duct disruption after laparoscopic cholecystectomy. *Semin Ultrasound CT MR* 1993; 14:346–355.

SECTION 4

The Gastrointestinal Tract

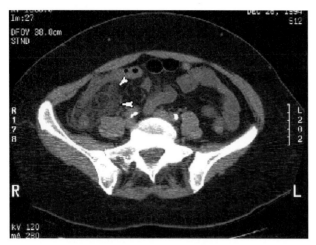

FIG. 61A. Non-contrast–enhanced CT

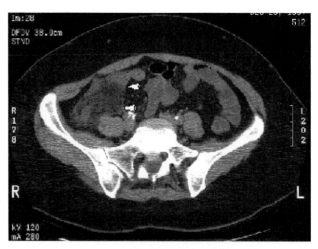

FIG. 61B. Non-contrast–enhanced CT

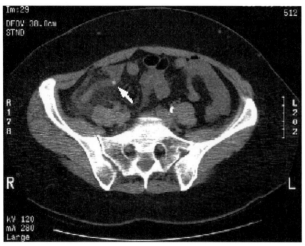

FIG. 61C. Non-contrast–enhanced CT

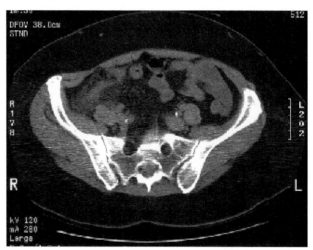

FIG. 61D. Non-contrast–enhanced CT

History

Right lower quadrant pain. Rule out appendicitis.

Findings

Figures 61A–D are non-contrast-enhanced spiral CT scans of the midabdomen and pelvis. In the right lower quadrant note the edema of the mesentery in all four images (arrowheads). A tubular structure representing a dilated appendix is identified in Figure 61C. In Figure 61C there is a calcified appendicolith at the base of the appendix (arrow).

Diagnosis

Acute appendicitis.

Discussion

The use of spiral CT without either intravenously or orally administered contrast enhancement for the diagnosis of appendicitis is somewhat controversial. In thin patients the minimally inflamed appendix may be extremely difficult to visualize without either orally or intravenously administered contrast medium. In obese patients, however, non-contrast-enhanced CT may offer some significant advantages when compared to sonography, since inflamed periappendiceal fat is much more readily appreciable. The calcified appendicolith in this patient was also clearly identified by CT. In patients with possible periappendiceal abscesses, intravenously contrast enhancement is useful to identify liquified areas of abscess formation. Phlegmonous masses will be of soft-tissue density.

References

Balthazar EJ, Birnbaum BA, Yee J, Megibow AJ, Roshkow J, Gray C. Acute appendicitis: CT and US correlation in 100 patients. *Radiology* 1994; 190:31–35.

Balthazar EJ, Megibow AJ Siegel SE, Birnbaum BA. Appendicitis: prospective evaluation with high-resolution CT. *Radiology* 1991; 180:21–24.

Malone AJ Jr, Wolf CR, Malmed AS, Melliere BF. Diagnosis of acute appendicitis: value of unenhanced CT. *AJR* 1993; 160:763–766.

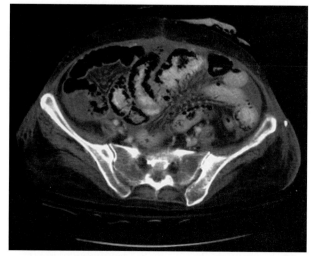

FIG. 62A. Contrast-enhanced CT

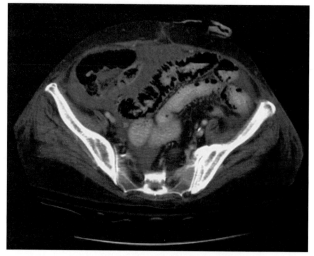

FIG. 62B. Contrast-enhanced CT

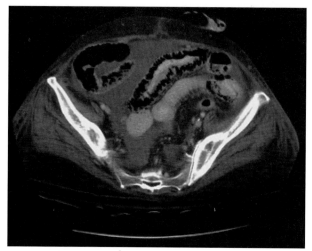

FIG. 62C. Contrast-enhanced CT

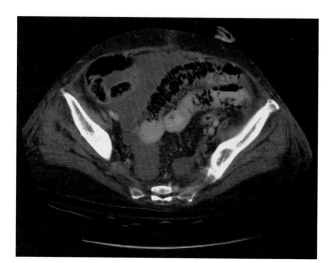

FIG. 62D. Contrast-enhanced CT

History

Increasing abdominal pain following laparotomy for lysis of adhesions. Rule out small bowel obstruction.

Findings

Figures 62A–D are contrast-enhanced spiral CT scans of the midabdomen and pelvis. Note that throughout all four images there is moderate ascites as well as extensive pneumatosis of the distal small bowel.

Diagnosis

Small-bowel infarction.

Discussion

At surgery, 5 feet of necrotic ileum was resected. A definitive cause of small-bowel infarction was not proven, since both the superior mesenteric artery and vein were patent at the time of surgery. It is likely that a postoperative low-flow state resulted in intestinal ischemia. Spiral CT is an excellent modality for evaluating luminal abnormalities of the gastrointestinal tract. Because of a lack of misregistration artifacts occurring in breath-hold imaging, paging through serial CT sections often demonstrates subtle gastrointestinal-tract pathology not detectable by dynamic CT. In this patient the pneumatosis was obvious and due to bowel infarction. Benign causes of pneumatosis (e.g., chronic obstructive pulmonary disease, bowel resection) should always be kept in mind. The clinical course of the patient is a very important indicator in determining the need for surgery.

References

Grieshop RJ, Dalsing MC, Cikrit DF, Lalka SG, Sawchuk AP. Acute mesenteric venous thrombosis. Revisited in a time of diagnostic clarity. *Am Surg* 1991; 57:573–577.

Smerud MJ, Johnson CD, Stephens DH. Diagnosis of bowel infarction: a comparison of plain films and CT scans in 23 cases. *AJR* 1990; 154:99–103.

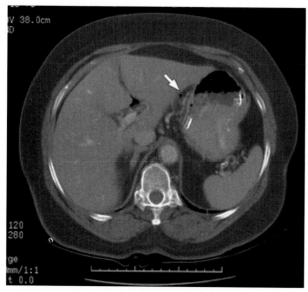

FIG. 63A. Contrast-enhanced CT

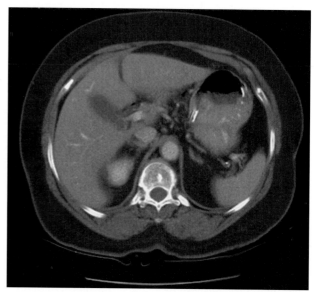

FIG. 63B. Contrast-enhanced CT

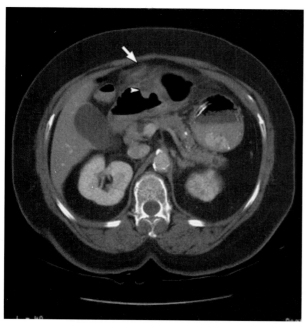

FIG. 63C. Contrast-enhanced CT

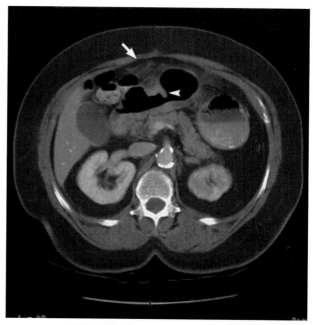

FIG. 63D. Contrast-enhanced CT

History

Midepigastric pain. Rule out abscess.

Findings

Figures 63A–D are contrast-enhanced spiral CT scans of the upper abdomen performed with a single breath-hold. Notice in Figure 63A and B the small amount of pneumoperitoneum seen adjacent to the gastrohepatic ligament (arrow) and the porta hepatis. Figures 63C and D demonstrate soft-tissue infiltration of the omentum (arrow) and mural thickening of the stomach (arrowhead).

Diagnosis

Perforated gastric ulcer.

Discussion

The patient's clinical presentation mimicked an abscess, owing to the presence of spiking fevers and upper abdominal pain. Because of the ability to perform breath-hold imaging without misregistration artifacts, the tiny gas bubbles of pneumoperitoneum were clearly identified in this patient. Although most commonly seen in the upper abdomen in the anterior subphrenic spaces, pneumoperitoneum from gastrointestinal-tract perforations may be trapped by upper abdominal ligaments, such as the gastrohepatic ligament or the hepatoduodenal ligament. Endoscopy revealed a large, lesser-curvature ulcer that was benign. The patient was treated conservatively without surgery, and made a relatively uneventful recovery with broad-spectrum antibiotics.

References

Fultz PJ, Skucas J, Weiss SL. CT in upper gastrointestinal tract perforations secondary to peptic ulcer disease. *Gastrointest Radiol* 1992; 17:5–8.

Ranschaert E, Rigaute H. Confined gastric perforation: ultrasound and computed tomographic diagnosis. *Abdom Imag* 1993; 18:318–319.

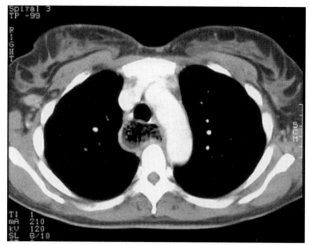

FIG. 64A. Contrast-enhanced CT

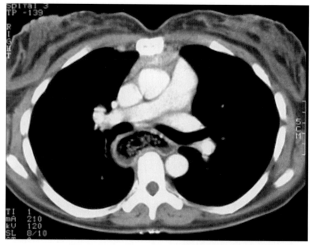

FIG. 64B. Contrast-enhanced CT

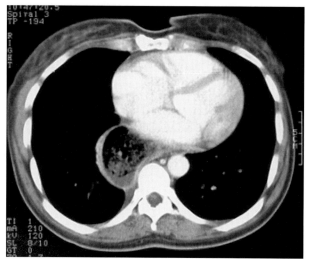

FIG. 64C. Contrast-enhanced CT

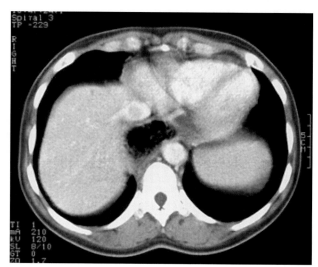

FIG. 64D. Contrast-enhanced CT

History

A 40-year-old female with a widened mediastinum on a chest radiograph. A spiral CT scan was ordered to rule out a possible mass.

Findings

A spiral CT scan demonstrated a markedly dilated esophagus with a moderate amount of food and fluid matter within it. The esophageal wall measured less than 1 cm in thickness at all levels evaluated. The patient had no evidence of focal mass in the esophagus. The dilatation extended down to the esophageogastric junction, with no site of obstruction. The esophagus was subsequently biopsied.

Diagnosis

Achalasia of the esophagus.

Discussion

Achalasia is a rare motor disorder of the esophagus resulting in aperistalsis of the lower esophagus and inadequate relaxation of the lower esophageal sphincter. Achalasia occurs in the general population with an incidence of 0.6 to 2 cases per 100,000 patients per year. In most cases the diagnosis of achalasia is made prior to a CT scan being obtained, although in other cases, such as the one presented, CT may be the initial study to suggest the diagnosis. Although achalasia is usually diagnosed and evaluated with either barium swallow or endoscopy, CT can provide valuable information in indeterminate cases, or reveal the presence of this disease in patients evaluated for other causes of mediastinal widening.

In the patient with known achalasia, there are several potential applications for CT. They include evaluation of potential complications of therapy, including iatrogenic esophageal perforation or pulmonary aspiration. A fistula between the esophagus and trachea may also be detected. Since there is increased incidence of carcinoma in patients with achalasia, CT can also be the initial study to suggest the presence of esophageal cancer and to determine its extent. The proven incidence of carcinoma of the esophagus in patients with achalasia runs as high as 20%, although the typical figure quoted is around 7%. If the patient indeed has esophageal cancer, then in addition to CT, an evaluation by magnetic resonance imaging (MRI) may be helpful.

The differential diagnosis of the CT appearance of achalasia includes esophageal stricture due to inflammatory or neoplastic disease. However, it would be improbable to see such dilatation proximal to a stricture related to inflammatory or neoplastic disease without the patient being symptomatic. Also, in these cases there is diffuse esophageal thickening, typically at the level of narrowing, while in achalasia this has not been the case in our experience.

References

Cassela RR, Brown AL Jr, Sayre GGP, Ellis FH Jr. Achalasia of the esophagus: pathologic and etiologic considerations. *Ann Surg* 1964; 160:474–487.

Rabushka LS, Fishman EK, Kuhlman JE. CT evaluation of achalasia. *J Comput Assist Tomogr* 1991; 15:434–439.

Rosenzweig S, Traube M. The diagnosis and misdiagnosis of achalasia. A study of 25 consecutive patients. *J Clin Gastroenterol* 1989; 11:147–153.

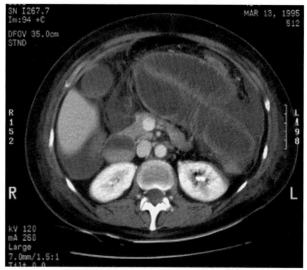

FIG. 65A. Contrast-enhanced CT

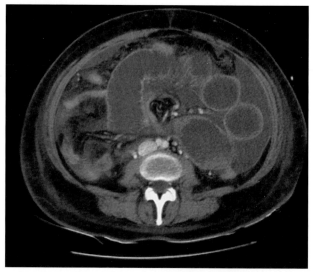

FIG. 65B. Contrast-enhanced CT

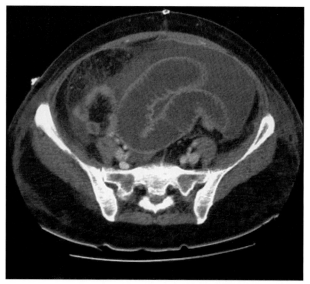

FIG. 65C. Contrast-enhanced CT

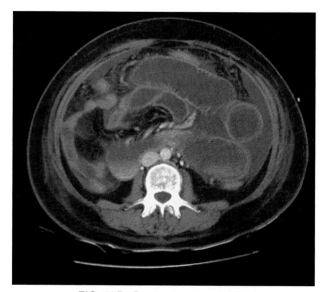

FIG. 65D. Contrast-enhanced CT

History

Persistent abdominal pain following gastric surgery.

Findings

Figures 65A–D are contrast-enhanced spiral CT scans of the mid- and lower abdomen. Note the marked dilatation of the small bowel with associated free intraperitoneal fluid. In Figure 65D several loops of distal and small bowel are collapsed.

Diagnosis

Small-bowel obstruction.

Discussion

The plain abdominal radiographs, both supine and upright, were negative in this patient. This was because the dilated small bowel was completely filled with fluid and there were no air–fluid levels. The CT diagnosis of small-bowel obstruction is based primarily on the identification of a transitional zone between dilated and nondilated bowel. Unusual causes of small-bowel obstruction, such as intussusception, closed-loop obstruction, or neoplasms obstructing the bowel can be clearly diagnosed with CT. The advantage of spiral CT is that the lack of misregistration artifact through breath-hold imaging affords rapid paging through the entire data set to visualize the course of the bowel longitudinally. The transition between dilated and nondilated bowel is more readily appreciated in this scanning mode.

References

Balthazar EJ, George W. Holmes Lecture. CT of small-bowel obstruction. *AJR* 1994; 162:255–261.
Frager D, Medwid SW, Baer JW, Mollinelli B, Friedman M. CT of small-bowel obstruction: value in establishing the diagnosis and determining the degree and cause. *AJR* 1994; 162:37–41.

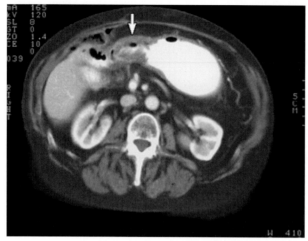

FIG. 66A. Contrast-enhanced CT

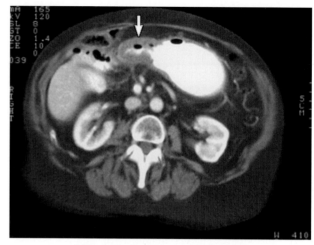

FIG. 66B. Contrast-enhanced CT

History

A 70-year-old female who had undergone Whipple's procedure for pancreatic cancer. The patient had adjuvant radiation therapy to the tumor bed. A spiral CT was done for routine follow-up.

Findings

A spiral CT scan demonstrates thickening of the wall of the gastric antrum. The gastric antrum measured about 10 mm in thickness (arrow).

Diagnosis

Radiation gastritis.

Discussion

Spiral CT is an ideal method for detecting pancreatic pathology as well as for evaluating the patient who has undergone pancreatic surgery. In the patient with pancreatic cancer, Whipple's procedure is the only treatment modality that could result in long-term survival, since there is currently no chemotherapy that is successful in pancreatic cancer. However, successful surgery requires removal of all tumor; microscopic tumor spread may be present even if surgical margins are negative. Postoperative adjuvant therapy typically includes radiation therapy, which is routinely part of the therapeutic regimen in many institutions. The most important use of CT as a monitoring study in this group of patients is to distinguish between changes related to therapy and changes related to tumor recurrence. Spiral CT, because of its excellent opacification of vasculature and the ability to obtain narrow interscan intervals, is the study of choice for following these patients.

Radiation gastritis occurs most commonly in patients who receive doses exceeding 50 Gy (5000 rad) over a 5-week period. This condition is typically seen between 1 month and 2 years after therapy. As in the present case, thickening of the gastric wall is most commonly seen in the area of the gastro-jejunostomy, corresponding to the peak focus of irradiation.

The CT and pathologic findings of radiation gastritis are fairly consistent. Thickening of the gastric wall is often seen in a symmetric pattern in patients who have had therapy for pancreatic cancer. Small ulcerations may be seen in the mucosa, and the CT picture may be described as "shaggy." Pathologically, injury to the epithelium of the stomach results in mucosal ulcerating and sloughing. Frank ulceration may occur, depending on the extent of associated vascular injury. One of the key points of recognizing radiation gastritis is to not confuse it with recurrent or residual tumor, although in select cases the appearance of the two may be identical. In our experience, most patients with CT evidence of radiation gastritis do not have clinical symptomatology, although some may present with delayed gastric emptying or in more severe cases with gastric outlet obstruction.

References

Bluemke DA, Fishman EK, Kuhlman JE, Zinreich ES. Complications of radiation therapy: CT evaluation. *RadioGraphics* 1991; 11:581–600.

Henry G. Emphysematous gastritis. *AJR* 1952; 68:15–18.

Williamson MR, Shah HR, Harper RR, Angtuaco TL. CT of emphysematous gastritis. *Comput Med Imag Graph* 1989; 13(2):175–177.

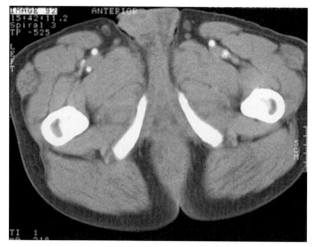

FIG. 67A. Contrast-enhanced CT

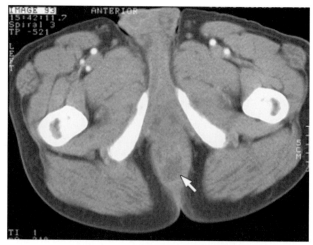

FIG. 67B. Contrast-enhanced CT

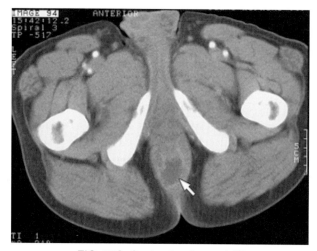

FIG. 67C. Contrast-enhanced CT

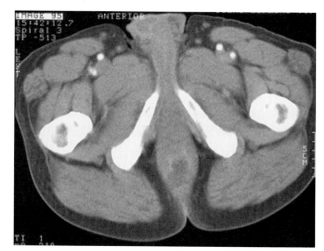

FIG. 67D. Contrast-enhanced CT

History

A 42-year-old human immunodeficiency virus (HIV)-positive male with a history of increasing perirectal pain, including pain on defecation.

Findings

The study demonstrates evidence of a fluid collection in the left perirectal region (arrow) within the levator ani muscle. There are minimal inflammatory changes present in the ischiorectal fossa.

Diagnosis

Perirectal abscess.

Discussion

Perirectal inflammatory disease is most commonly associated with a variety of inflammatory processes including inflammatory bowel disease, such as Crohn disease, radiation proctitis, and proctitis in homosexual male patients.

With the increased use of CT in the evaluation of the HIV-positive patient, we are seeing more cases of perirectal inflammatory disease. Spiral CT can be done by using a caudal-to-cranial scanning direction following the intravenous infusion of contrast material. This technique allows excellent discrimination of vessels and distinction of vessels from potential nodal masses. It also allows a careful analysis in both transaxial and multiplanar display of the perirectal region, including the ischiorectal fossa and lower pelvis.

Guillaumin et al. have reported their findings in 42 patients with perirectal inflammatory disease and suspected perirectal abscess. They found that CT was reliable for distinguishing perirectal abscess from cellulitis, and for localizing abscesses in both the supralevator and infralevator regions. They note that one of the advantages of CT is in revealing a supralevator abscess that might be missed on surgical exploration unless the surgeons look carefully for it. CT would undoubtedly help guide the surgeon in such cases.

In general, spiral CT is advantageous in the pelvis because of the ability to acquire data at maximum vascular enhancement. In cases in which the pelvis is the primary area of interest, we will either start inferiorly, at the level just beneath the symphysis pubis, and scan cranially, or begin at the iliac crest and scan caudally. There does not appear to be a significant difference in the results with either protocol.

References

Bevans DW. Perirectal abscess: a potentially fatal illness. *Am J Surg* 1973; 126:765–768.

Guillaumin E, Jeffrey RB Jr, Shea WJ, Asling CW, Goldberg HI. Perirectal inflammatory disease: CT findings. *Radiology* 1986; 161:153–157.

Pozniak M, Petasnick JP, Matalon TAS, Bayard WJ. Computed tomography in the differential diagnosis of pelvic and extrapelvic disease. *RadioGraphics* 1985; 5:587–610.

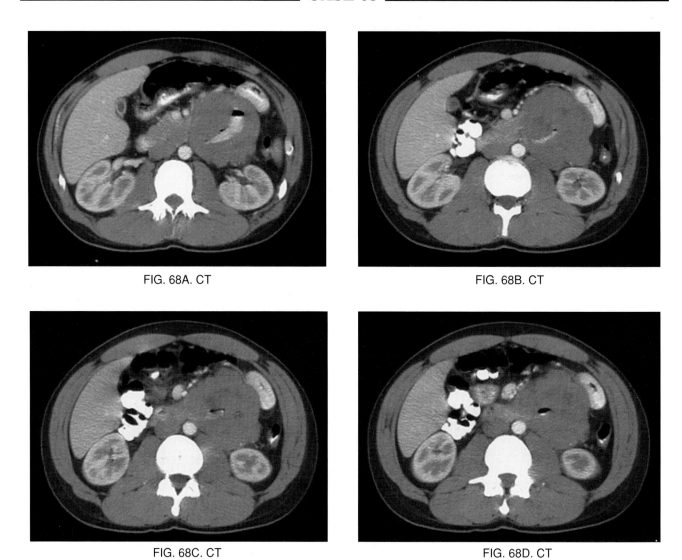

FIG. 68A. CT

FIG. 68B. CT

FIG. 68C. CT

FIG. 68D. CT

History

A 29-year-old male presented with a history of fever, chills, fatigue, and right-upper-quadrant pain increasing over several months. Spiral CT was done for evaluation.

Findings

A spiral CT scan demonstrates a 7-cm mass involving the proximal jejunum, with encasement and ulceration. The tumor extends to near the superior mesenteric artery and vein, but does not appear to involve them. Displacement of mesenteric vessels is seen.

Diagnosis

Non-Burkitt's lymphoma of the small bowel.

Discussion

The use of spiral CT may be important both in detecting small bowel pathology and in its differential diagnosis. In the present case, the clear definition of the tumor mass in relationship to adjacent vascular structures is well documented. In addition, the mass has areas of necrosis but does not enhance.

The differential diagnosis in this case would include a leiomyosarcoma, lymphoma, or adenocarcinoma. If this were indeed a leiomyosarcoma, we would expect enhancement on a spiral CT. Leiomyosarcomas will enhance by about 1.5 times the baseline value because of their vascularity. The bulkiness of the tumor mass in this case would tend to suggest that it does not represent adenocarcinoma but more likely a lymphoma. This was indeed the case at biopsy.

Spiral CT, in addition to diagnosing tumor mass, is an excellent in defining the extent of tumor. Two- and three-dimensional images can also be obtained and can be used if radiation therapy is the treatment modality of choice.

Small-bowel lymphomas can be divided into several categories based either on their radiologic appearance or pathology. The radiologic differentiation includes infiltrating tumor, polypoid-mass-type tumors, multifocal nodules with or without intussusception, ulcerating masses, and eccentric masses.

References

Clark RA, Alexander ES. Computed tomography of gastrointestinal leiomyosarcoma. *Gastrointest Radiol* 1984; 7:127–129.

Dudiak KM, Johnson CD, Stephens DH. Primary tumors of the small intestine: CT evaluation. *AJR* 1989; 52:995–998.

Megibow AJ, Balthazar EJ, Naidich DP. Computed tomography of gastrointestinal lymphoma. *AJR* 1983; 141:541–547.

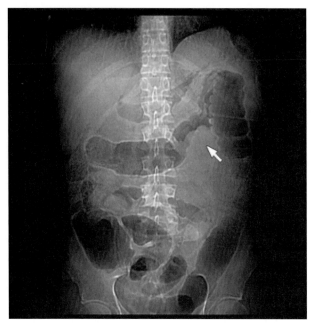

FIG. 69A. Digital scout radiograph

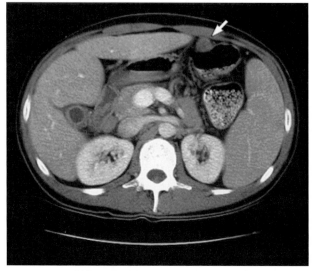

FIG. 69B. Contrast-enhanced CT

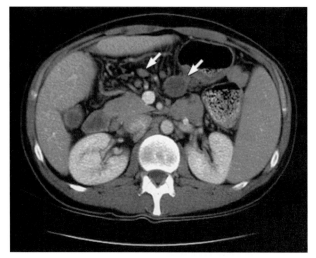

FIG. 69C. Contrast-enhanced CT

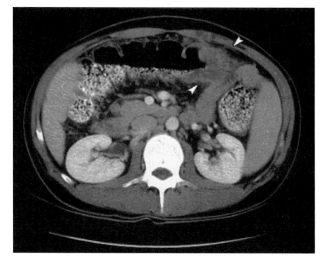

FIG. 69D. Contrast-enhanced CT

History

A 40-year-old male with a 20-year history of ulcerative colitis. Now with increasing abdominal pain.

Findings

Figure 69A is a digital scout radiograph of the abdomen demonstrating focal narrowing of the distal transverse colon (arrow). Figures 69B–D are contrast-enhanced scans from a spiral CT. Note in Figure 69B the serosal implant along the anterior wall of the stomach. In Figure 69C there are multiple enlarged mesenteric lymph nodes (arrows) adjacent to a thickened segment of distal transverse colon. One lymph node measures approximately 2 cm in size. Figure 69D demonstrates marked mural thickening of the transverse colon (arrowheads).

Diagnosis

Colon carcinoma with peritoneal and nodal metastases.

Discussion

This patient's colon carcinoma was associated with a long-standing history of ulcerative colitis. At the time of presentation, the lesion was already metastatic to the peritoneum and adjacent mesenteric lymph nodes. The spiral CT scan in this patient clearly demonstrated the serosal implant on the anterior wall of the body of the stomach, as well as the multiple enlarged mesenteric lymph nodes. No liver metastases were detected either on the preoperative spiral CT or with intraoperative ultrasonography.

References

McGahren ED 3rd, Mills SE, Wilhelm MC. Colorectal carcinoma in patients 30 years of age and younger. *Am Surg* 1995; 61:78–82.

Megibow AJ. "Computed tomography and magnetic resonance imaging in colorectal carcinoma: staging and detection of postoperative recurrence." In: PC Freeney, GW Stevension (eds.): *Margulis and Burhenne's Alimentary Tract Radiology*, 5th ed. St. Louis: OV Mosby, 1994, pp. 801–810.

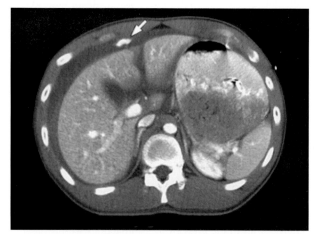

FIG. 70A. Contrast-enhanced CT

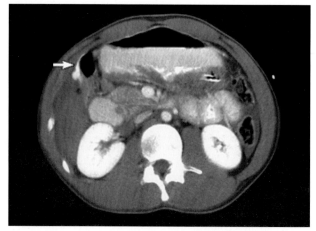

FIG. 70B. Contrast-enhanced CT

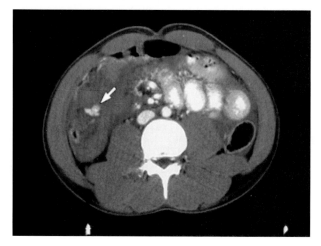

FIG. 70C. Contrast-enhanced CT

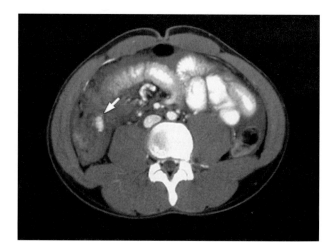

FIG. 70D. Contrast-enhanced CT

History

A patient who had been involved in a motor vehicle accident, with abdominal pain and a falling hematocrit.

Findings

Figures 70A–D are contrast-enhanced spiral CT scans of the abdomen. Note in Figure 70A and B hemoperitoneum surrounding the liver and extending into the right paracolic gutter. Note a high-density focus anterior to the left hepatic lobe, representing active arterial extravasation (arrow). In Figure 70B, this can be seen to originate from a gastroepiploic vessel adjacent to the distal antrum and duodenum. Figures 70C and D demonstrate another site of active arterial extravasation (arrow), from the mesentery of the right colon. Notice a large hematoma in the adjacent mesentery. There is a focal area of high attenuation, isodense with the adjacent aorta, that is consistent with active arterial extravasation. Several small-bowel loops seen in the midabdomen show evidence of bowel-wall thickening consistent with edema and contusion.

Diagnosis

Multiple sites of active arterial extravasation due to blunt abdominal trauma.

Discussion

Active arterial extravasation is a critical observation in patients undergoing spiral CT for blunt abdominal trauma. This finding necessitates either immediate surgery or angiographic embolization; as conservative therapy is unwarranted. Areas of active arterial extravasation have the typical features of: (1) high-attenuation foci similar in density to major adjacent arterial structures; and (2) a large surrounding hematoma.

At times, highly attenuating active arterial extravasation may be confused with extravasated orally administered contrast material. However, a large hematoma generally displaces bowel, and should be a feature discriminating these two entities from one another. At surgery multiple sites of active bleeding were noted, and a right colectomy was required to control bleeding.

References

Jeffrey RB Jr, Cardoza JD, Olcott EW. Detection of active intraabdominal arterial hemorrhage: value of dynamic contrast-enhanced CT. *AJR* 1991; 156:725–729.

O'Sullivan G, Williams M, Hughes PM. Mesenteric arterial rupture following blunt abdominal trauma: demonstration by computed tomography (letter). *Br J Radiol* 1994; 67:1143–1144.

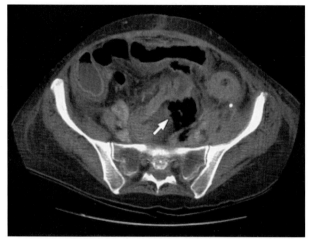

FIG. 71A. Contrast-enhanced CT

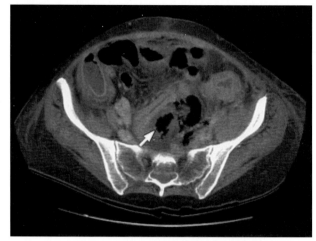

FIG. 71B. Contrast-enhanced CT

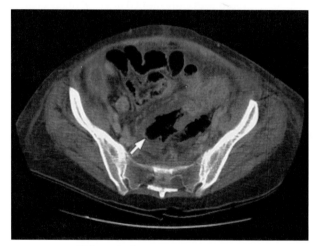

FIG. 71C. Contrast-enhanced CT

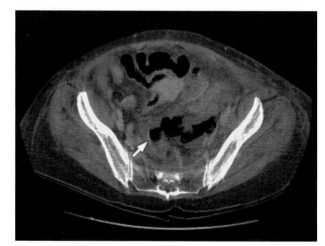

FIG. 71D. Contrast-enhanced CT

History

Fever and septicemia following cardiac surgery. The patient had been receiving intravenous antibiotics for pneumonia for 2 weeks.

Findings

Figures 71A–D are contrast-enhanced spiral CT scans of the pelvis. Note in Figure 71A and B the excellent opacification of the mucosal surface of the right colon. There is extensive mural thickening and edema of the colon. In addition, ectopic gas is seen adjacent to the sigmoid colon on all four images (arrow).

Diagnosis

Pseudomembranous colitis with perforation of the sigmoid colon.

Discussion

Sepsis and colonic perforation were the predominant findings in this patient's clinical presentation of pseudomembranous colitis. Often there is a more benign clinical course, with fever and diarrhea. However, this is not invariably the case. Some are diagnostic dilemmas, presenting with fever of unknown origin without diarrhea. In febrile patients receiving antibiotics, the presence of colonic wall thickening on CT should always raise a suspicion of pseudomembranous colitis. Titers of antibody to *Clostridium difficile* should be obtained. When these are positive, appropriate antibiotic therapy (generally vancomycin) can be initiated, often with excellent results. However, in this patient the diagnosis was not made prior to colonic perforation with ectopic gas seen in the sigmoid mesentery.

References

Boland GW, Lee MJ, Cats AM, Gaa JA, Saini S, Mueller PR. Antibiotic-induced diarrhea: specificity of abdominal CT for the diagnosis of Clostridium difficile disease. *Radiology* 1994; 191:103–106.

Fekety, Shah AB. Diagnosis and treatment of Clostridium difficile colitis. *JAMA* 1993; 269:71–75.

Fishman EK, Kavuru M, Jones B. Pseudomembranous colitis: CT evaluation of 26 cases. *Radiology* 191; 180:57–60.

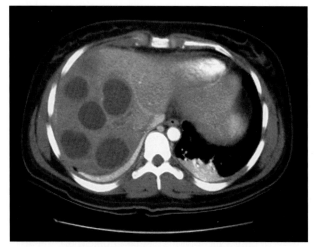

FIG. 72A. Contrast-enhanced CT liver

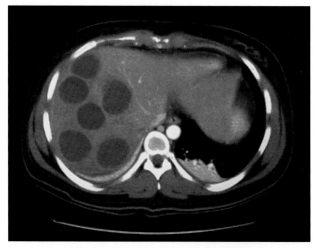

FIG. 72B. Contrast-enhanced CT liver

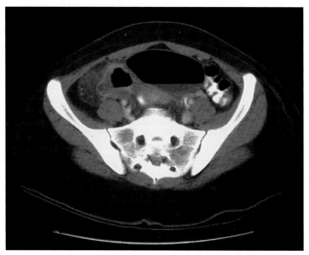

FIG. 72C. Contrast-enhanced CT pelvis

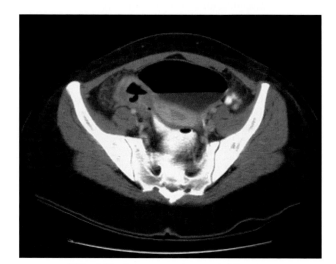

FIG. 72D. Contrast-enhanced CT pelvis

History

A 19-year-old female with pelvic pain and fever.

Findings

Figures 72A and B are spiral CT scans of the liver obtained following intravenous infusion of contrast medium. Note the multiple, rounded, low-density lesions clustered together in the right lobe of the liver. Figures 71C and D are scans of the pelvis demonstrating an air–fluid level in the bladder and an adjacent gas-containing mass representing an abscess.

Diagnosis

Crohn's disease of the sigmoid colon, complicated by a colovesical fistula and multiple pyogenic liver abscesses.

Discussion

The multiple low-density hepatic lesions in this patient were "clustered" in a pattern that is typical for pyogenic liver abscesses. This was probably due to portal venous bacteremia from the patient's pelvic abscess. The abscess was due to Crohn's disease of the sigmoid colon, with extension into the bladder. The air–fluid level in the bladder was diagnostic of a colovesical fistula.

References

Barrada R, Ros PR. Diagnostic imaging of liver abscess. *Crit Rev Diagn Imag* 1992; 33:29–58.

Georges RN, Deitch EA. Pyogenic hepatic abscess. *South Med J* 1993; 86:1233–1235.

Hochbergs P, Forsberg L, Hederstrom E, Andersson R. Diagnosis and percutaneous treatment of pyogenic hepatic abscesses. *Acta Radiol* 1990; 31:351–353.

Jeffrey RB Jr, Tolentino CS, Chang FC, Federle MP. CT of small pyogenic hepatic abscesses: the cluster sign. *AJR* 1988; 151:487–489.

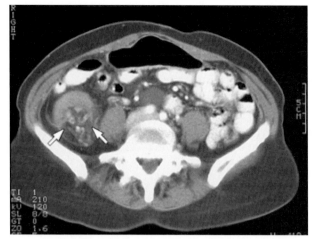

FIG. 73A. Contrast-enhanced CT

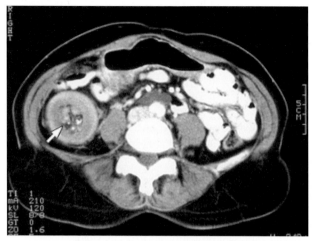

FIG. 73B. Contrast-enhanced CT

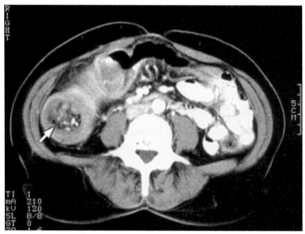

FIG. 73C. Contrast-enhanced CT

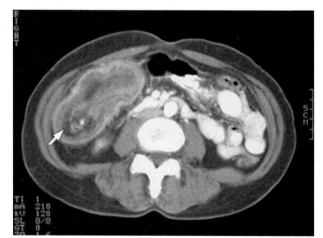

FIG. 73D. Contrast-enhanced CT

History

This 66-year-old female with a history of anemia and gastrointestinal bleeding had a barium enema, which suggested a mass in the cecum. A CT scan was ordered for staging prior to operative resection of the mass.

Findings

A spiral CT scan demonstrates the classic appearance of an intussusception involving the bowel in the right lower quadrant. On cross section, we can clearly see the crescent of fat along with the vascular structures, which are enhancing and which extend through the midportion of the intussusception (arrows). The mass has intussuscepted all the way up and into the midportion of the transverse colon. Interestingly, the patient's small bowel appeared unremarkable, and there was no small-bowel obstruction or ileus.

Diagnosis

Adenocarcinoma of the cecum intussuscepting into the colon to the proximal transverse colon.

Discussion

The role of CT in the evaluation of the patient with suspected or known colon cancer is typically for the staging of disease by revealing the presence or absence of extracolonic disease. The presence of liver metastases, adenopathy, or carcinomatosis obviously has a major impact on the therapy chosen by the physician, particularly when a more extensive resection is necessary. CT has been used in attempts to stage the depth of invasion of tumor. The results have been mixed despite adherence to very strict scanning protocols, including colonic distension with air.

Spiral CT does have the advantage of vascular opacification of the smaller pelvic vessels, thereby helping to discriminate between small nodes and normal vasculature. Gazelle et al. used an enema for colonic distension in an attempt to analyze the depth of tumor invasion and local extension in a series of 30 patients. They found that 23 of the patients were staged correctly. Of those patients incorrectly staged, four were understaged and three were overstaged. Interestingly, all cases of incorrect staging involved in predicting lymph node involvement. One limitation that persists even with spiral CT is that node size remain essentially the sole criterion for determining whether a node is benign or malignant. Organ-specific contrast agents such as EOE-13 have not been successfully produced in large quantities, and the radiologic pharmaceutical manufacturers have not been successful in developing a new reticuloendothelial system agent. Finally, the intussusception in this case is somewhat interesting in that the patient was asymptomatic despite the CT appearance. Many intussusceptions seen on CT are intermittent, and the radiologic and clinical findings may not directly correlate.

References

Buetow PC, Buck JL, Carr NJ, Pantongrag-Brown L. From the Archives of the AFIP. Colorectal adenocarcinoma: radiologic-pathologic correlation. *RadioGraphics* 1995; 15:127–146.

Gazelle GS, Gaa J, Saini S, Shellito P. Staging of colon carcinoma using water enema CT. *J Comput Assist Tomogr* 1995; 19(1):87–91.

Padidar AM, Jeffrey RB Jr, Mindelzun RE, Dolph JF. Differentiating sigmoid diverticulitis from carcinoma on CT scans: mesenteric inflammation suggests diverticulitis. *AJR* 1994; 163:81–83.

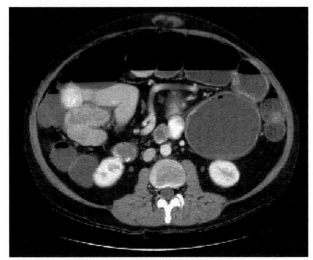

FIG. 74A. Contrast-enhanced CT

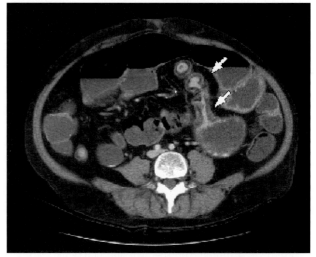

FIG. 74B. Contrast-enhanced CT

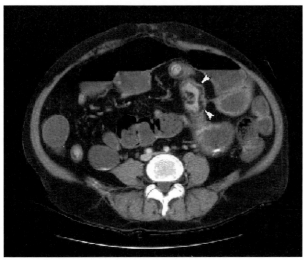

FIG. 74C. Contrast-enhanced CT

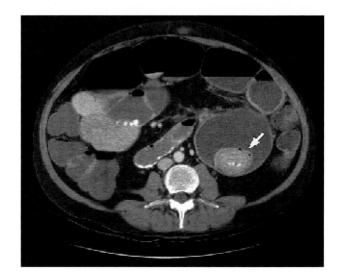

FIG. 74D. Contrast-enhanced CT

History

Crohn's disease with increasing abdominal pain.

Findings

Figures 74A–D are contrast-enhanced spiral CTs of the midabdomen. Note that in all four images there is marked dilatation of the small bowel. In Figure 74A a small umbilical hernia is identified. In Figure 74B and C there is an abrupt transition zone from dilated to nondilated bowel (arrows, Figure 74B). Notice also the mural thickening of the stenotic segment of bowel. Submucosal fat deposition is present in the stenotic segment, compatible with Crohn's disease (arrowheads, Figure 74C). A large calcified enterolith caused by chronic high-grade, partial small-bowel obstruction is identified (arrow, Figure 74D).

Diagnosis

Chronic small-bowel obstruction secondary to Crohn's disease.

Discussion

In this patient, the cause of the small-bowel obstruction was Crohn's disease. A calcified enterolith developed within a segment of bowel proximal to a chronic low-grade obstruction. Submucosal fat deposition is quite characteristic of inflammatory bowel disease and can be seen, particularly in the colon, in cases of ulcerative colitis and Crohn's disease. In selective patients it may also be noted in the small bowel. This patient ultimately underwent surgical resection of the diseased segment of the small bowel, which demonstrated stenotic Crohn's disease.

References

Manakawa S, Takahashi M, Takagi K, Takano M. The role of computed tomography in management of patients with Crohn disease. *Clin Imag* 1993; 17:193–198.

Megibow AJ, Balthazar EJ, Cho KC, Medwid SW, Birnbaum BA, Noz ME. Bowel obstruction: evaluation with CT. *Radiology* 1991; 180:313–318.

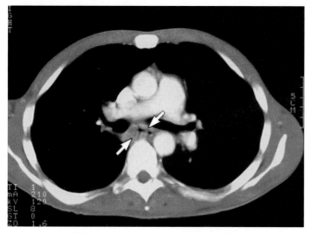

FIG. 75A. Contrast-enhanced CT

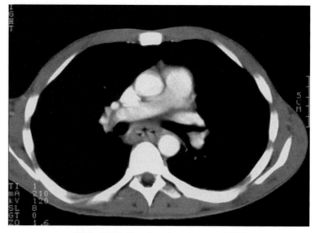

FIG. 75B. Contrast-enhanced CT

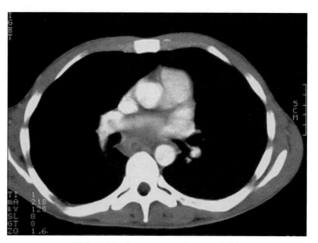

FIG. 75C. Contrast-enhanced CT

History

A 33-year-old male who was human immunodeficiency virus (HIV)-positive, with a low CD4 cell count. Routine chest x-ray suggested a mediastinal mass. Spiral CT was done for evaluation.

Findings

A spiral CT scan shows no evidence of a tumor mass in the mediastinum or hilar regions. The scan did, however, demonstrate marked thickening of the esophagus (arrows), with the extent of involvement being nearly the entire distal two-thirds of the esophagus. This pattern is most consistent with an inflammatory process, although a superimposed neoplasm cannot be excluded based solely on the CT examination. No evidence of mediastinal abscess or adenopathy is present.

Diagnosis

Esophagitis due to candidiasis and *Mycobacterium avium* infection.

Discussion

The CT evaluation of the patient with acquired immune deficiency syndrome (AIDS) is a common examination in most large-city hospitals. The AIDS patient is subject to a wide range of inflammatory and neoplastic conditions, which is particularly true for patients with low CD4 cell counts. Gastrointestinal manifestations are common and can involve any portion of the gastrointestinal tract. Opportunistic infections could be caused by viral, fungal, protozoan, or bacterial pathogens. Patients with AIDS also have increased incidence of primary tumors of the gastrointestinal tract, including Kaposi sarcoma and non-Hodgkin lymphoma.

CT is usually not the study that is first performed in the patient with esophagitis. However, with the increased use of CT for AIDS patients and with CT being the primary modality for evaluation of the mediastinum, it is not surprising that esophagitis can be detected. The most common cause of infectious esophagitis is *Candida* infection, which is thought to result from the downward spread of the fungus from the oropharynx to the esophagus. Deep esophageal ulceration, intramural dissection, or fistula formation may occur, but the picture is more suggestive of an infection such as tuberculosis than of *Candida* infection. Although *Candida* is the most common agent, other agents that involve the esophagus in the AIDS patient include cytomegalovirus (CMV), herpes simplex virus, and *Mycobacterium avium* complex (MAI). In fact, in many AIDS patients a single isolated pathogen will not be detected; rather, multiple pathogens will be detected at the same time. In the present case, both candidiasis and *Mycobacterium avium* infection were present in the biopsy specimen.

Spiral CT with thin sections and close interscan spacing is also excellent at defining potential complications of esophagitis, which include large ulcerations, perforation, and secondary abscess formation. One limitation of CT, even with spiral mode, is that it can be difficult if not impossible to distinguish between esophagitis and carcinoma based simply on their CT appearance. In both cases, the esophagus will appear thickened in either a symmetric or asymmetric pattern. However, the clinical history as well as secondary findings may be helpful. We have rarely seen adenopathy in patients with esophagitis, while it is a common occurrence in the patient with carcinoma.

References

Kuhlman JE, Fishman EK, Wang K, Siegelman SS. Esophageal duplication cyst: CT and transesophageal needle aspiration. *AJR* 1985; 145:531–532.

Noh HM, Fishman EK, Forastiere AA, Bliss DF, Calhoun PS. CT of the esophagus: spectrum of disease. *RadioGraphics* 1995; 15:1113–1134.

Pantongrag-Brown L, Nelson AM, Brown AE, Buetow PC, Buck JL. Gastrointestinal manifestations of acquired immunodeficiency syndrome: radiologic-pathologic correlation. *RadioGraphics* 1995; 15:1155–1178.

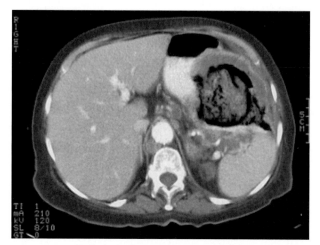

FIG. 76A. Contrast-enhanced CT

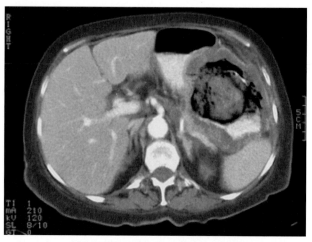

FIG. 76B. Contrast-enhanced CT

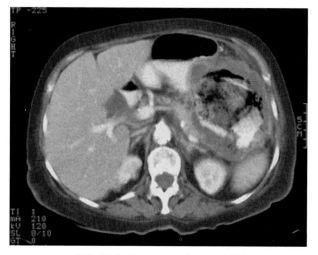

FIG. 76C. Contrast-enhanced CT

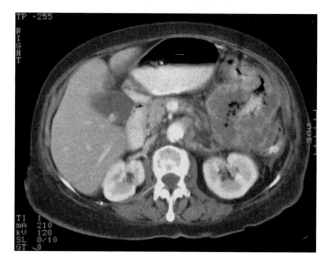

FIG. 76D. Contrast-enhanced CT

History

A 73-year-old female with a history of abdominal pain and foul-smelling breath. The clinical history also suggested possible episodes of bowel obstruction.

Findings

A spiral CT scan demonstrates an approximately 10-cm ulcerating mass in the left upper quadrant, involving the stomach and region of the splenic flexure. There are no clear planes between the ulcerating mass and the pancreas and spleen. Subcrural nodes are also seen. The differential diagnosis in this case centers on a possible sarcoma arising from the stomach or a mass arising from the colon. The possibility of a retroperitoneal mass extending forward or a large mass arising from or near the pancreas would also have to be considered.

Diagnosis

Gastrocolic fistula due to ulcerating carcinoma of the transverse colon.

Discussion

Although initially felt to be a problem-solving tool to be used in select cases, spiral CT has become the standard examination in the evaluation of abdominal pathology.

In the present case, the study clearly demonstrates a large ulcerating mass as well as defining the extent of involvement. Although one cannot be 100% specific about the etiology of this mass, the information necessary for the surgeon, both with regard to the local extent of disease and distant metastases such as to lymph nodes, is clearly defined. In fact, our initial interpretation of the scan was that the mass probably arose from the stomach and represented an ulcerating leiomyosarcoma with local extension. It was somewhat to our surprise that the primary pathology was a colonic lesion, considering that the patient had no evidence of obstruction on the CT scans.

Spiral CT is a key study in the evaluation of patients with colon cancer. We have recently reviewed a series of 21 patients with metastatic disease to the liver, with close correlation of surgical and pathologic findings. We found that for lesions over 1 cm in size, spiral CT had approximately a 91% accuracy in lesion detection. This study was based on portal venous phase imaging only. This is comparable with statistics noted for CTAP CT and better than the standard reported accuracies for magnetic resonance imaging (MRI).

Hollett et al. noted that with a dual-phase spiral CT there is even a further increase in lesion detection, of just under 10%. Therefore, it is our feeling that dual-phase spiral CT of the liver in patients with metastatic disease will have a far better than 90% detection rate. Consequently, this should be the standard modality for evaluating these patients.

The most common cause of gastrocolic fistula is a neoplasm. This is true for either a gastric cancer eroding through the mesocolon into the transverse colon, or, as in the present case, a large colonic cancer invading the stomach. Other, less common causes of gastrocolic fistulas include iatrogenic perforation or perforation by a foreign body. Fistulization by inflammatory conditions, including diverticulitis and inflammatory bowel disease, should also be considered in an extensive differential diagnosis.

References

Hollett MD, Jeffrey RB Jr, Nino-Murcia M, Jorgensen MJ, Harris DP. Dual phase helical CT of the liver: Value of arterial phase scans in the detection of small (≤1.5 cm) malignant hepatic neoplasms. *AJR* 1995; 164:879–884.

Kusyzk BS, Bluemke DA, Urban BA, Choti MA, Hruban RH, Sitzmann JV, Fishman EK. Portal-phase contrast-enhanced helical CT for the detection of malignant hepatic tumors; sensitivity based on comparisons with intraoperative and pathologic findings. *AJR* 1996;166:91–95.

Scatarige JC, Fishman EK, Jones B, Cameron JL, Sanders RC, Siegelman SS. Gastric leiomyosarcoma: CT observations. *J Comput Assist Tomogr* 1985; 9:320–327.

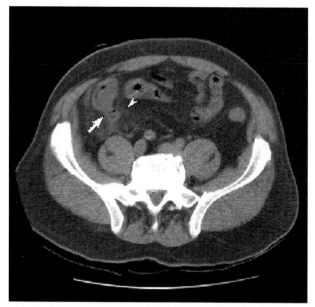

FIG. 77A. Non-contrast–enhanced CT

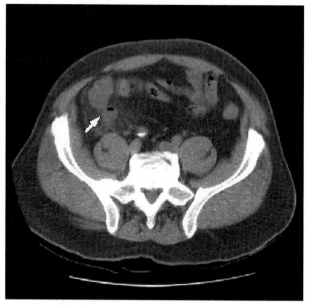

FIG. 77B. Non-contrast–enhanced CT

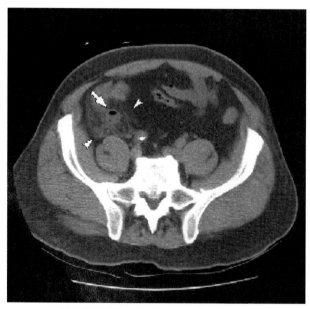

FIG. 77C. Non-contrast–enhanced CT

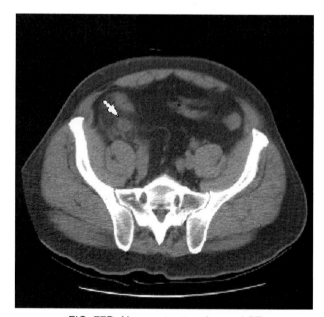

FIG. 77D. Non-contrast–enhanced CT

History

Right lower quadrant pain. Rule out appendicitis.

Findings

Figures 77A–D are spiral CT scans of the right lower quadrant performed without either oral or intravenous administration of contrast material. Notice the edema and soft-tissue infiltration around the cecum (arrowheads) and appendix. The appendix contains gas (arrows) and is located just medial to the tip of the cecum.

Diagnosis

Appendicitis with a gas-containing appendix.

Discussion

In patients with significant intraperitoneal fat, non-contrast-enhanced CT scans can be useful for evaluating the right lower quadrant for suspected appendicitis. Oral and intravenous administration of contrast medium are most helpful when scanning thin patients without significant mesenteric or omental fat. One of the most useful CT signs of appendicitis is periappendiceal edema. CT is most helpful when there is more advanced inflammation. Early acute, uncomplicated appendicitis may be very difficult to visualize by CT without intravenously administered contrast medium. This case was somewhat unusual in that the appendix contained gas. This was undoubtedly secondary to a gas-forming infection within the lumen.

Sonography is most helpful in normal size adult women and in thin males. Sonography excels in revealing gynecologic pathology and for evaluating for appendicitis in patients who are not obese. In obese patients or patients with suspected appendiceal perforation, spiral CT with intravenous and oral administration of contrast material is the technique of choice.

References

Balthazar EJ, Birnbaum BA, Yee J, Megibow AJ, Roshow J, Gray C. Acute appendicitis: CT and US correlation in 100 patients. *Radiology* 1994; 190:31–35.

Birnbaum BA, Balthazar EJ. CT of appendicitis and diverticulitis. *Radiol Clin North Am* 1994; 32:885–898.

Malone AJ Jr, Wolf CR, Malmed AS, Mellier BF. Diagnosis of acute appendicitis: value of unenhanced CT. *AJR* 1993; 160:763–766.

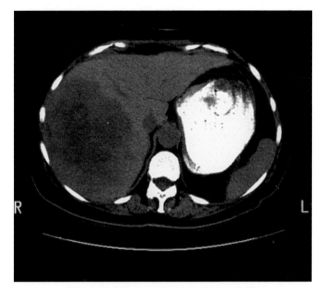

FIG. 78A. Non-contrast–enhanced CT

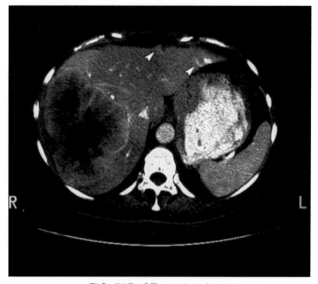

FIG. 78B. CT:arterial phase

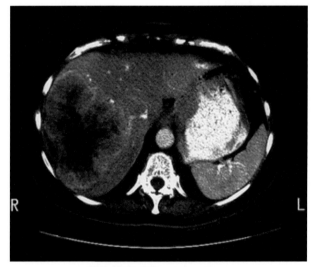

FIG. 78C. CT:venous phase

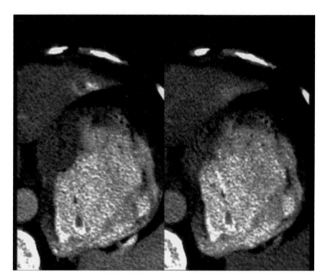

FIG. 78D. CT:arterial/venous phases

History

Colon carcinoma with rising CEA.

Findings

Figures 78A–D are scans obtained from a biphasic spiral CT of the liver. Figure 78A is a non-contrast-enhanced scan demonstrating a large, low-density lesion involving almost the entire right lobe. Figure 78B is an arterial-phase image demonstrating peripheral enhancement around the large right-lobe lesion, as well as rim enhancement around two additional lesions seen in the lateral segment of the left lobe (arrowheads). Figure 78C is a scan obtained during the portal venous phase, showing no evidence of the two left-lobe lesions. Figure 78D is a side-by-side comparison of the arterial and portal venous-phase images of the left lobe.

Diagnosis

Metastatic colon carcinoma to the liver. Left-lobe metastasis demonstrated only on arterial-phase images.

Discussion

The diagnostic yield of biphasic spiral CT for detection of liver metastases from colon cancer is relatively low. However, in this patient the lesions in the lateral segment were evident only on the arterial-phase images. Increased flow was seen around the periphery of the lesions. On portal venous-phase images, there was washout of contrast material and the lesions became nearly isodense with the surrounding liver. With greater experience it may be possible to more accurately predict which patients might benefit from biphasic spiral CT of the liver. Because of the increased radiation dose entailed by the dual acquisitions, and the more rapid injection rate (5 ml/sec) of contrast medium, this technique is not indicated in all patients with colon carcinoma. It may be useful, however, in patients when initial CT scans obtained only during the portal venous phase are equivocal.

References

Hollett MD, Jeffrey RB Jr, Nino-Murcia M, Jorgensen, MJ, Harris DP. Dual-phase helical CT of the liver: value of arterial phase scans in the detection of small (≤1.5 cm) malignant hepatic neoplasms. *AJR* 1995; 164:879–884.

Megibow AJ. "Computed tomography and magnetic resonance imaging in colorectal carcinoma: staging and detection of postoperative recurrence." In: PC Freeney, GW Stevenson (eds.). *Margulis and Burhenne's Alimentary Tract Radiology*, 5th ed. St. Louis: CV Mosby, 1994, pp. 801–810.

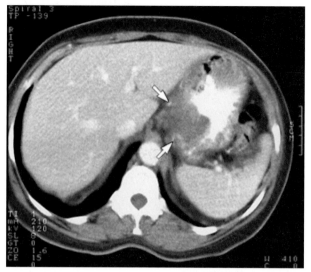

FIG. 79A. Contrast-enhanced CT

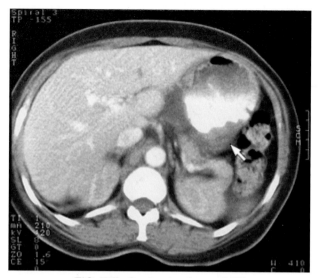

FIG. 79B. Contrast-enhanced CT

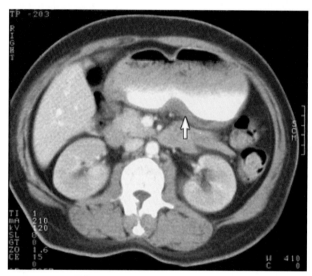

FIG. 79C. Contrast-enhanced CT

History

A 52-year-old female with a history of gastric ulcer disease and complaints of nausea, vomiting, and inability to retain food. The patient also experienced dull epigastric pain.

Findings

A spiral CT scan following distension of the stomach with 750 ml of positive oral contrast material demonstrates large lobular folds in the gastric fundus, with thickening of the posterior gastric wall, as well as at the level of the antrum (arrows). No evidence of adenopathy was seen.

Diagnosis

Helicobacter pylori gastritis simulating a gastric neoplasm.

Discussion

Helicobacter pylori is a gram-negative, spiral-shaped bacillus that is currently recognized as a worldwide pathogen. It is most commonly found beneath the mucus layer of surface epithelial cells, where it is commonly present in superficial foveolar cells in the stomach. The gastric antrum has been the most common site of involvement, although any area in the stomach may be involved. The prevalence of *H. pylori* increases with age, with more than 50% of Americans over 60 years of age being infected by this organism. However, only a small minority of patients are symptomatic. Much work has gone into study of the relationship between *H. pylori* and peptic ulcer disease and/or gastric carcinoma. Most articles suggest that there is an important relationship between gastric and duodenal ulcers and *H. pylori* infection. In some series, *H. pylori* has been found in up to 80% of patients with gastric ulcers and nearly 100% of patients with duodenal ulcers. Several studies have demonstrated a greater incidence of *H. pylori* in patients with gastric cancer than in the general population. In fact, at least one study has suggested that chronic *H. pylori* gastritis may be implicated in the development of gastric lymphoma. Although most cases of *H. pylori* gastritis are discovered on endoscopy, others can be discovered on radiographic imaging examinations. Sohn et al. recently compared double-contrast-enhanced upper gastrointestinal series in 88 patients with *H. pylori* and 41 control patients, and found that thickened gastric folds were detected in 44% of the patients with *H. pylori* and 9 of the control patients.

Urban et al. previously noted that on CT scanning there can be overlap between the appearance of *H. pylori* gastritis and gastric cancer. They retrospectively reviewed a series of 61 patients with biopsy-proven *H. pylori* gastritis. Of these studies, 19 patients had gastric abnormalities on CT, in 14 of whom the abnormalities were reported as suspicious for neoplasm. The two major patterns of severe *H. pylori* infection identified on CT were: (1) circumferential antral wall thickening; and (2) thickening of the posterior wall along the greater curvature, with or without evidence of ulceration. The thickening averaged 1.5 to 2 cm in cases suspicious for malignancy. The majority of abnormalities involved the gastric antrum. The important features that were not present were lack of significant adenopathy, obliteration of fat planes, or invasion of adjacent organs.

In the case presented here, the large thick folds in the gastric fundus and body were suggestive of an underlying neoplasm, with the differential diagnosis including adenocarcinoma or lymphoma. A biopsy was done in this patient, and revealed *H. pylori* infection. It is important for the radiologist to be aware of the potential confusion between this entity and a neoplasm, and to recognize that endoscopy may be necessary for a definitive diagnosis due to the overlap in their appearance.

References

Levine MS, Rubesin SE. The Helicobacter pylori revolution: Radiologic perspective. *Radiology* 1995; 195:593–596.

Sohn J, Levine MS, Furth EE, et al. Helicobacter pylori gastritis: radiographic findings. *Radiology* 1995; 195:763–767.

Urban BA, Fishman EK, Hruban RH. Helicobacter pylori gastritis mimicking gastric carcinoma at CT evaluation. *Radiology* 1991; 179:689–691.

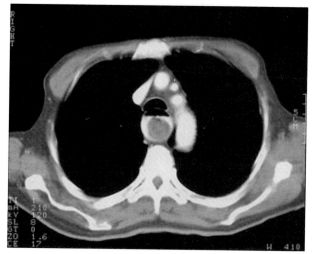

FIG. 81A. Contrast-enhanced CT

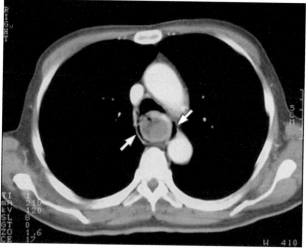

FIG. 81B. Contrast-enhanced CT

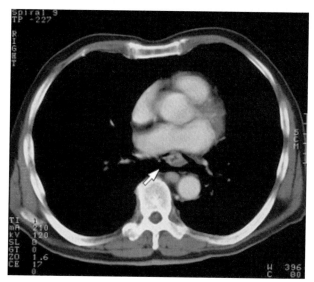

FIG. 81C. Contrast-enhanced CT

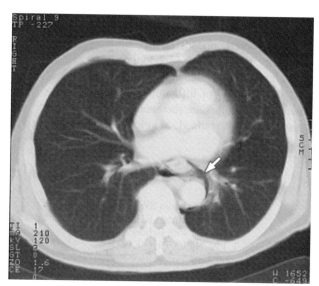

FIG. 81D. Contrast-enhanced CT

History

A 81-year-old male with a history of esophageal cancer. The patient was undergoing a laser procedure to decrease tumor bulk and keep the esophagus open.

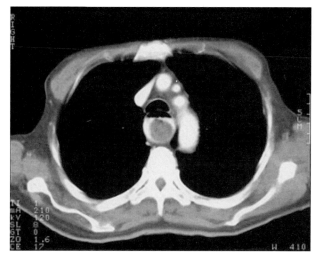

FIG. 81A. Contrast-enhanced CT

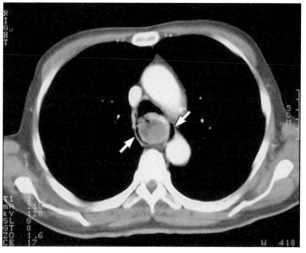

FIG. 81B. Contrast-enhanced CT

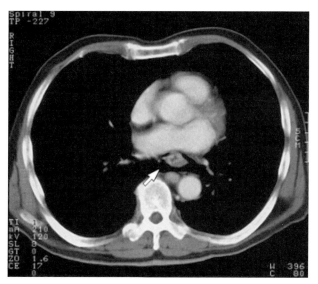

FIG. 81C. Contrast-enhanced CT

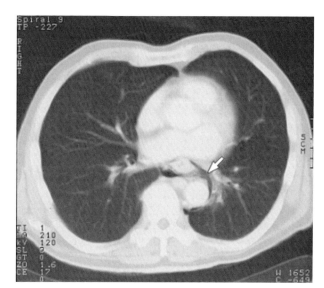

FIG. 81D. Contrast-enhanced CT

History

A 81-year-old male with a history of esophageal cancer. The patient was undergoing a laser procedure to decrease tumor bulk and keep the esophagus open.

Findings

CT demonstrated a lobulated soft-tissue mass in the root of the mesentery with a focus of calcification (arrow) within the mass. There appeared to be fingerlike projections extending from the mass toward the small bowel, which was slightly displaced. The CT appearance favored a carcinoid tumor, but other possibilities, including desmoid tumor, lymphoma, metastatic disease, or inflammatory disease of the mesentery, would have to be considered in the differential diagnosis.

Diagnosis

Inflammatory pseudotumor of the mesentery.

Discussion

The description of the mass and its CT appearance was most classic for carcinoid tumor, which was the presumptive diagnosis prior to biopsy. The presence of a focus of calcification truly enhanced the diagnosis of carcinoid tumor, particularly because of the irregularity of the mass and its fingerlike projections. As noted above for the differential diagnosis of mesenteric masses, an inflammatory process is also a possibility. Inflammatory pseudotumors are unusual benign entities that mimic malignancy in many different organ systems. The etiology of inflammatory pseudotumors is unknown. These tumors are mesenchymal growths composed of large, loosely arranged, nonpleomorphic spindle cells.

Inflammatory pseudotumors have been reported in the liver, spleen, kidney, pancreas, stomach, and bladder. In the cases described in the literature, inflammatory pseudotumors were impossible to distinguish radiographically from a primary malignant or metastatic process.

The present case is a good example of the ability of spiral CT to clearly defined the appearance and extent of a lesion, although without being 100% specific in terms of making the diagnosis. In the evaluation of mesenteric processes, spiral CT can play a major role by defining the true extent of disease and helping determine the logical sequence of events for making a definitive diagnosis.

References

Enzinger FM, Weiss SW. *Soft Tissue Tumors*, 2nd ed. St. Louis: CV Mosby, 1988, p. 210.

Pretorius ES, Hruban RH, Fishman EK. Inflammatory pseudotumor of the terminal ileum mimicking malignancy in a patient with Behcet's disease: CT and pathologic findings. *Clin Imag* (In press).

Shek TW, Ng IO, Chan KW. Inflammatory pseudotumor of the liver: report of four cases and review of the literature. *Am J Surg Pathol* 1993; 17:321–328.

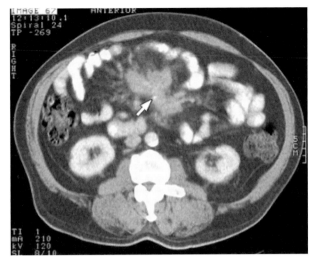

FIG. 80A. Contrast-enhanced CT

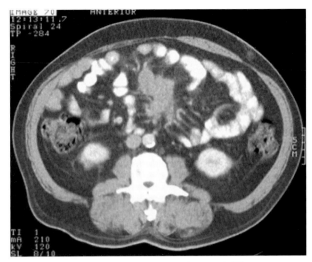

FIG. 80B. Contrast-enhanced CT

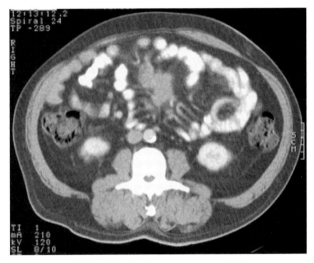

FIG. 80C. Contrast-enhanced CT

History

A 64-year-old male with abdominal pain and weight loss.

Findings

A spiral CT scan following distension of the stomach with 750 ml of positive oral contrast material demonstrates large lobular folds in the gastric fundus, with thickening of the posterior gastric wall, as well as at the level of the antrum (arrows). No evidence of adenopathy was seen.

Diagnosis

Helicobacter pylori gastritis simulating a gastric neoplasm.

Discussion

Helicobacter pylori is a gram-negative, spiral-shaped bacillus that is currently recognized as a worldwide pathogen. It is most commonly found beneath the mucus layer of surface epithelial cells, where it is commonly present in superficial foveolar cells in the stomach. The gastric antrum has been the most common site of involvement, although any area in the stomach may be involved. The prevalence of *H. pylori* increases with age, with more than 50% of Americans over 60 years of age being infected by this organism. However, only a small minority of patients are symptomatic. Much work has gone into study of the relationship between *H. pylori* and peptic ulcer disease and/or gastric carcinoma. Most articles suggest that there is an important relationship between gastric and duodenal ulcers and *H. pylori* infection. In some series, *H. pylori* has been found in up to 80% of patients with gastric ulcers and nearly 100% of patients with duodenal ulcers. Several studies have demonstrated a greater incidence of *H. pylori* in patients with gastric cancer than in the general population. In fact, at least one study has suggested that chronic *H. pylori* gastritis may be implicated in the development of gastric lymphoma. Although most cases of *H. pylori* gastritis are discovered on endoscopy, others can be discovered on radiographic imaging examinations. Sohn et al. recently compared double-contrast-enhanced upper gastrointestinal series in 88 patients with *H. pylori* and 41 control patients, and found that thickened gastric folds were detected in 44% of the patients with *H. pylori* and 9 of the control patients.

Urban et al. previously noted that on CT scanning there can be overlap between the appearance of *H. pylori* gastritis and gastric cancer. They retrospectively reviewed a series of 61 patients with biopsy-proven *H. pylori* gastritis. Of these studies, 19 patients had gastric abnormalities on CT, in 14 of whom the abnormalities were reported as suspicious for neoplasm. The two major patterns of severe *H. pylori* infection identified on CT were: (1) circumferential antral wall thickening; and (2) thickening of the posterior wall along the greater curvature, with or without evidence of ulceration. The thickening averaged 1.5 to 2 cm in cases suspicious for malignancy. The majority of abnormalities involved the gastric antrum. The important features that were not present were lack of significant adenopathy, obliteration of fat planes, or invasion of adjacent organs.

In the case presented here, the large thick folds in the gastric fundus and body were suggestive of an underlying neoplasm, with the differential diagnosis including adenocarcinoma or lymphoma. A biopsy was done in this patient, and revealed *H. pylori* infection. It is important for the radiologist to be aware of the potential confusion between this entity and a neoplasm, and to recognize that endoscopy may be necessary for a definitive diagnosis due to the overlap in their appearance.

References

Levine MS, Rubesin SE. The Helicobacter pylori revolution: Radiologic perspective. *Radiology* 1995; 195:593–596.

Sohn J, Levine MS, Furth EE, et al. Helicobacter pylori gastritis: radiographic findings. *Radiology* 1995; 195:763–767.

Urban BA, Fishman EK, Hruban RH. Helicobacter pylori gastritis mimicking gastric carcinoma at CT evaluation. *Radiology* 1991; 179:689–691.

Findings

A spiral CT scan demonstrates a dilated upper esophagus with an air–fluid level. There also appears to be air present around the esophagus (arrows), consistent with perforation. Extension of air down the posterior mediastinum is also noted. No evidence of pleural effusion is seen.

Diagnosis

Esophageal perforation following laser therapy in a patient with esophageal cancer.

Discussion

Spiral CT is commonly requested for patients who have had an endoscopic or interventional procedure that has or may have resulted in a complication. Endoscopic evaluation of the esophagus or upper airway can result in numerous complications, including that of esophageal perforation. Esophageal perforation is potentially a life-threatening event. Although perforation is usually diagnosed by classic signs and symptoms including vomiting, chest pain, fever, and subcutaneous emphysema, in other cases radiologic studies are necessary. Bladergroen et al. reviewed 114 cases of esophageal rupture and found that the perforation was iatrogenic in 55%. The majority of patients in the study had underlying disease including strictures, achalasia, or cancer.

CT scanning does have several advantages when used for diagnosing esophageal perforation. White et al. reviewed 12 cases of esophageal perforation and found abnormalities including esophageal thickening (9 patients), paraesophageal fluid (11 patients), extraluminal air (11 patients), and pleural effusion (9 patients). The CT scan is very sensitive to the presence of air, and even minimal amounts of air in the mediastinum can easily be detected.

We previously reviewed 18 cases of iatrogenic rupture of the esophagus. In cervical esophageal rupture (four cases), findings included pneumomediastinum (three cases), posterior mediastinal abscess (one case), tracheoesophageal fistula (one case), and small bilateral pleural effusions (two cases). In rupture of the thoracic esophagus (10 cases), findings included free extravasation to the left pleural space (3 cases), contained extravasation (7 cases), bilateral pleural effusions (9 cases), isolated left pleural effusion (1 case), and pneumomediastinum (3 cases). All patients with free extravasation required surgery, whereas all patients with contained thoracic esophageal extravasation were treated conservatively.

Spiral CT also has the advantage of providing sequentially timed images with narrow interscan spacing. In these cases, subtle perforations may be detected and the extent of involvement defined. The role of spiral CT in these patients is to determine the extent of injury and whether or not patients can be managed conservatively or will need to undergo surgical repair. In many cases of esophageal perforation, watchful waiting tends to yield a successful outcome. On a technical note, our routine for evaluating the esophagus is to use Esopho-CAT (E-Z-EM, New York, NY) paste. This can be used with caution in a patient with possible perforation, to help define the presence and extent of a fistula.

References

Bladergroen MR, Lowe JE, Postlethwait RW. Diagnosis and recommended management of esophageal perforation and rupture. *Ann Thorac Surg* 1986; 42:235–239.

Halden WJ, Harnsberger HR, Mancuso AA. Computed tomography of esophageal varices after sclerotherapy. *AJR* 1986; 147:57–60.

Noh HM, Fishman EK, Forastiere AA, Bliss DF, Calhoun PS. CT of the esophagus: spectrum of disease with emphasis on esophageal carcinoma. *RadioGraphics* 1995; 15:1113–1134.

The Genitourinary Tract

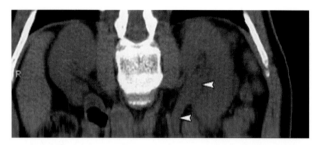

FIG. 82A.Oblique coronal non-contrast–enhanced CT

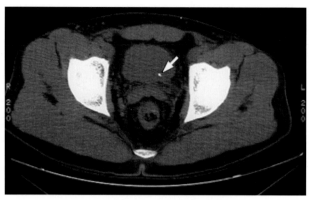

FIG. 82B. Axial non-contrast–enhanced CT

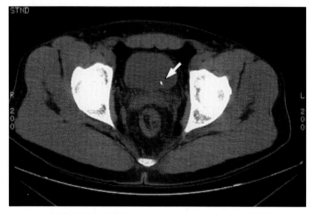

FIG. 82C. Axial non-contrast–enhanced CT

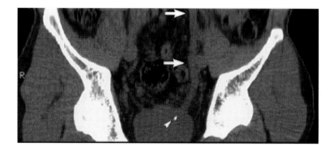

FIG. 82D. Coronal non-contrast–enhanced CT

History

Left flank pain. Rule out ureteral calculus.

Findings

Figures 82A–D are non-contrast-enhanced spiral CT scans of the abdomen and pelvis. Figure 82A is an oblique coronal view of the abdomen demonstrating hydronephrosis of the left kidney (arrowheads) with a small amount of perirenal fluid. Figures 82B and C are axial scans of the pelvis. Note a calcific density (arrow) near the left ureterovesical junction. Figure 82D is a coronal reformation through the plane of the left ureter, demonstrating the distal left calculus (arrowhead) and moderate left hydroureter (arrows).

Diagnosis

Left ureteral calculus.

Discussion

Non-contrast-enhanced spiral CT offers a number of advantages when compared to intravenous urography for the evaluation of patients with suspicious acute flank pain. It is superior to urography for identifying ureteral calculi, and is as accurate as urography in diagnosing hydronephrosis. Spiral CT can be performed in a matter of minutes. In patients with high-grade ureteral obstruction, it may take hours to opacify the distal ureter with excretory urography. Coronal reformations are particularly valuable in distinguishing ureteral calculi from other pelvic calcifications such as phleboliths.

References

Levin E. Acute renal and urinary tract disease. *Radiol Clin North Am* 1994; 32:989–1004.
Smith RC, Rosenfield AT, Choe KA, et al. Acute flank pain: comparison of non-contrast-enhanced CT and intravenous urography. *Radiology* 1995; 194:789–794.

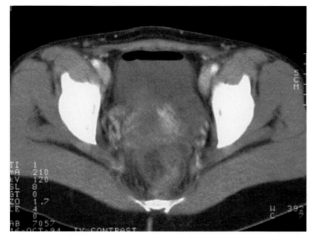

FIG. 83A. Contrast-enhanced CT

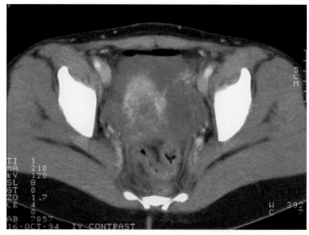

FIG. 83B. Contrast-enhanced CT

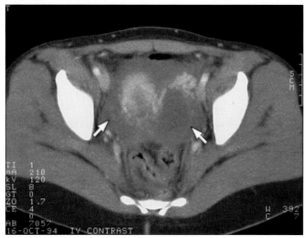

FIG. 83C. Contrast-enhanced CT

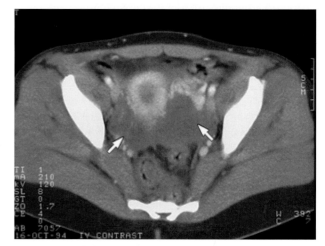

FIG. 83D. Contrast-enhanced CT

History

A 37-year-old female with a history of increasing lower abdominal and pelvic pain. The presumed clinical diagnosis is acute appendicitis. The differential diagnoses include endometriosis, pelvic inflammatory disease, and a ruptured ovarian cyst.

Findings

A spiral CT scan done in a caudal-to-cranial direction demonstrates bilateral cystic adnexal masses with septations. There is also minimal fluid in the pelvis.

Diagnosis

Ruptured endometriosis.

Discussion

In most patients, spiral CT is the study of choice for evaluation of the acute abdomen, because of its high sensitivity and specificity for a wide range of pathologic processes. For example, CT has a high sensitivity and specificity for the evaluation of suspected appendicitis. Although most patients with suspected appendicitis do not get CT scans, a CT scan is valuable for the rapid diagnosis and triage of patients in whom the diagnosis is questionable or the possibility of other pathology is suggested.

In the present case, a spiral CT scan was obtained, with the main clinical suspicion being appendicitis, but other possibilities were entertained. In fact, the cystic pelvic masses in this case were consistent with the diagnosis of endometriosis, which was part of the patient's past medical history. CT features of appendicitis were not seen.

Endometriosis affects a significant portion of the menstruating female population. It is estimated that 15% of all women will have this disease at some time during their reproductive lives. Most patients are in the age range of 20 to 40 years, and many are nulliparous. The symptoms have been described as dysmenorrhea, dyspareunia, and infertility. Although endometriosis can be asymptomatic in some patients, it can also mimic processes including pelvic inflammatory disease, urinary tract disease, and bowel disease. There has not been extensive CT literature on endometriosis. Those articles that have appeared have noted that endometriosis can be confused with other pathologies, including carcinoma or an infected ovarian cyst. Similarly, in the gastroenterology literature, articles have described how, on a barium enema, endometriosis can simulate a constricting lesion due to carcinoma.

With the increased use of CT, it is important for the radiologist to be aware of the possibility of endometriosis, especially in a patient with a history of atypical pelvic pain and cystic pelvic masses on CT.

References

Fishman EK, Scatarige JC, Saksouk FA, Rosenshein NB, Siegelman SS. Computed tomography of endometriosis. *J Comput Assist Tomogr* 1983; 7(2):257–264.
Heneghan MA, Texidor HS. Pleuroperitoneal endometriosis. *AJR* 1979; 133:727–730.
Schlueter FJ, McClennan BL. Massive ascites and pleural effusions associated with endometriosis. *Abdom Imag* 1994; 19:475–476.

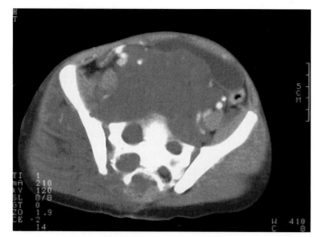

FIG. 84A. Contrast-enhanced CT

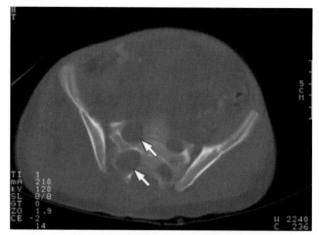

FIG. 84B. Contrast-enhanced CT

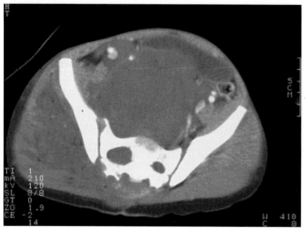

FIG. 84C. Contrast-enhanced CT

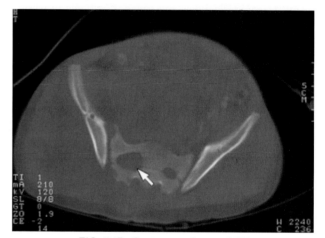

FIG. 84D. Contrast-enhanced CT

History

A 10-year-old male with a history of neurofibromatosis. CT was done to determine the extent of involvement.

Findings

A spiral CT scan demonstrates extensive bony changes in the pelvis with widening of the sacral foramina. There is a large presacral mass as well as multiple masses in the paraspinal muscles and in the region of the gluteal muscles in the right hemipelvis. This is consistent with widespread neurofibromatosis.

Diagnosis

Neurofibromatosis.

Discussion

Neurofibromatosis, or von Recklinghausen disease (VRN), is a disease characterized by neurofibromas involving multiple organs and organ systems. It is hereditary, with a dominant transmission in more than 50% of cases. CT scanning demonstrates a spectrum of appearances of neurofibromas, both in terms of extent and degree of involvement. Erosion of the sacral foramina with widening of the foramen is one of the most common findings. Kumar et al. previously reviewed a series of extracranial nerve-sheath tumors, including eight cases of neurofibromatosis. The authors noted varying attenuation values, and found hypodense lesions not to be uncommon. Several causes for the low density of neurofibromas include a population of lipid-rich Schwann cells, the presence of adipocytes in neurofibromas, and entrapment of perineuroadipose tissue by plexiform neurofibromas.

Neurofibromatosis may have the potential to degenerate into sarcomatous lesions. Neurofibrosarcomas are typically aggressive, with areas of necrosis and destruction. The terminology used to describe malignant transformation of neurofibromatosis includes neurofibrosarcoma, neurogenic sarcoma, and malignant schwannoma.

References

Biondetti PR, Vigo M, Fiore D, De Faveri D, Ravasini R, Benedetti L. CT appearance of generalized von Recklinghausen neurofibromatosis. *J Comput Assist Tomogr* 1983; 7:866–869.

Coleman BG, Arger PH, Dalinka MK, Obringer AC, Raney BR, Meadows AT. CT of sarcomatous degeneration in neurofibromatosis. *AJR* 1983; 140:383–387.

Kumar AJ, Kuhajda FP, Martinez CR, Fishman EK, Jezic DV, Siegelman SS. Computed tomography of extracranial nerve sheath tumors with pathological correlation. *J Comput Assist Tomogr* 1983; 7:857–865.

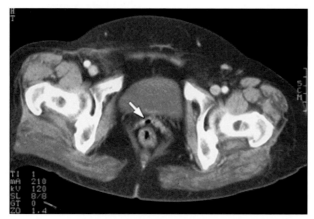

FIG. 85A. Contrast-enhanced CT

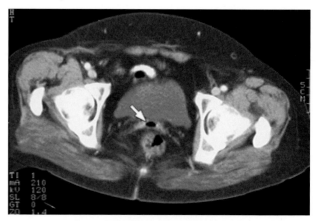

FIG. 85B. Contrast-enhanced CT

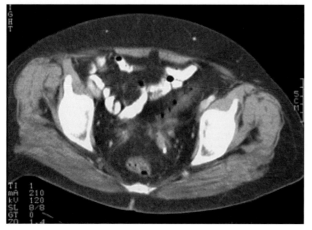

FIG. 85C. Contrast-enhanced CT

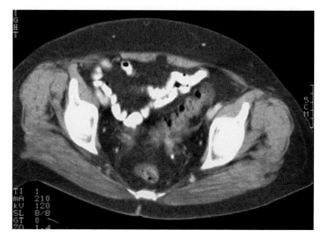

FIG. 85D. Contrast-enhanced CT

History

A 65-year-old female with a history of prior hysterectomy. The patient had recently been noted to be passing stool through the vagina.

Findings

Sequential spiral CT scans through the pelvis demonstrate air within the vagina. Evidence of diverticular disease is seen, with apparent fistulization between the colon and vagina.

Diagnosis

Enterovaginal fistulae.

Discussion

Spiral CT evaluation of the pelvis is valuable for a wide range of pelvic pathologies. In the present case, the study demonstrates air in the vagina, consistent with a fistula. CT scanning has been shown to be very accurate in detecting the site and cause of fistulae such as the one in this case. The presence of air in the vagina is an unusual finding. Nokes et al. previously reviewed 200 female cases to assess the frequency and significance of air in the vagina. Small amounts of air were not uncommonly seen on one section, and occurred in 11% of patients. Distention of the vagina with air or visualization of air in more than one image was typically seen only in patients with enterovaginal fistulae.

Enterovaginal fistulae are uncommon. The causes are variable, although diverticulitis, as in the present case, is responsible for nearly half of cases. Other causes include previous hysterectomy, Crohn disease, colon cancer, radiation to the pelvis, prior surgery, and perforation by a foreign body.

As has been noted in cases of enterovesical fistula, barium enema is an insensitive diagnostic technique, with less than a 50% success rate for detection. Scanning with spiral CT, which combines thin sections and narrow interscan collimation, should be very accurate in evaluating for the presence and cause of enterovaginal fistulae.

References

Craig O. Intestino-vaginal fistulae. *Br J Radiol* 1973; 46:48–53.

Nokes SR, Martinez CR, Arrington JA, Dauito R. Significance of vaginal air on computed tomography. *J Comput Assist Tomogr* 1986; 10(6):997–999.

Zeigerman JH, Stahlgren L, Tulsky EG. Sigmoidovaginal fistulas. Review of the literature and report of a case. *Am J Obstet Gynecol* 1964; 89:1003–1008.

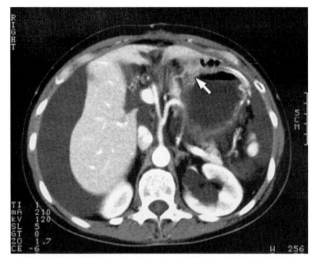

FIG. 86A. Contrast-enhanced CT

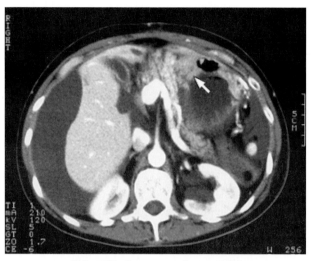

FIG. 86B. Contrast-enhanced CT

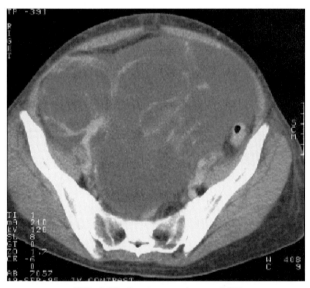

FIG. 86C. Contrast-enhanced CT

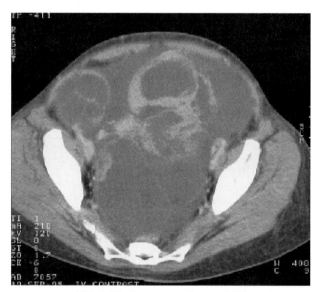

FIG. 86D. Contrast-enhanced CT

History

A 58-year-old female with a history of gastric adenocarcinoma and increasing abdominal girth.

Findings

A spiral CT scan with water as a contrast agent demonstrates evidence of focal thickening, with enhancement at the level of the gastrojejunostomy site (arrow). Extensive ascites is also present. On scans through the pelvic region, multiple large cystic pelvic masses are noted.

Diagnosis

Recurrent adenocarcinoma with malignant ascites and Krukenberg tumors.

Discussion

There has always been some controversy about the role of CT scanning in the evaluation of gastric cancer. A wide range of results have been reported, depending upon the specific series of patients reviewed. Part of the problem has been related to the techniques used, since many of the reported studies used older generation scanners and nonspiral techniques. With the introduction of spiral CT, there has been an increased interest in evaluation of the stomach.

In terms of technique, a recent study by Cho et al. combined gastric distention with water and intravenous bolus injection of contrast material. The technique used 600 to 800 ml of water and a 5 ml/sec injection of 150 ml of contrast material. A two-phase acquisition was obtained, with 30 seconds representing the early phase and 2 minutes representing the equilibrium phase. In this study, dynamic CT was used, rather than spiral CT. Despite this, and the fact that 10-mm-thick sections were used, Cho et al. were able to detect the primary tumors in 5 of 9 cases of early gastric cancer with a high degree of accuracy, and 41 of 43 cases of more advanced cancer, for an overall detection rate of 88%. This suggests that with spiral CT a high accuracy is possible for staging gastric cancer.

Similarly, in the patient with gastric adenocarcinoma following resection, spiral CT is an ideal study. In addition to a high degree of accuracy in detecting nodes in the region of the celiac axis, and the presence of liver metastases, the technique can clearly define potential recurrence at the anastomosis site, as in the present case. In appears that in cases of focal thickening at the anastomosis site, recurrent tumor will in part enhance.

It is also important that the entire abdomen and pelvis be scanned in the patient with gastric cancer, since the disease may spread distally to the uterus and ovary. In this case, large, complex, cystic and solid masses of the ovaries are seen, consistent with Krukenberg tumors.

The use of water as a contrast agent is being shown to be especially important in the evaluation of the stomach if one is to detect subtle disease, whether it is a primary or recurrent tumor. With positive contrast enhancement, this may be difficult to evaluate, particularly if one is looking for a change in the enhancement pattern of the gastric wall.

Finally, in this case, spiral CT and a properly timed injection provided excellent vascular opacification which is necessary if three-dimensional angiography is desired.

References

Cho J, Kim J, Rho S, Jeong H, Lee C. Preoperative assessment of gastric carcinoma: value of two-phase dynamic CT with mechanical IV injection of contrast material. *AJR* 1994; 163:69–75.

Hori S, Tsuda K, Murayama S, Matsushita M, Yukawa K, Kozuka T. CT of gastric carcinoma: preliminary results with a new scanning technique. *RadioGraphics* 1992; 12:257–268.

Minami M, Kawauchi N, Itai Y, Niki T, Sasaki Y. Gastric tumors: radiologic-pathologic correlation and accuracy of T-staging with dynamic CT. *Radiology* 1992; 185:173–178.

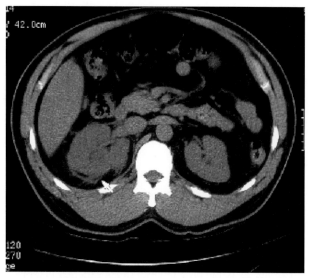

FIG. 87A. Non-contrast–enhanced CT

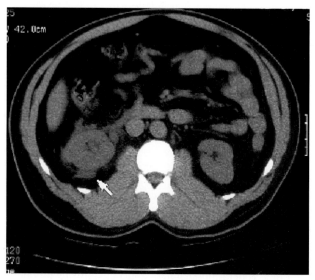

FIG. 87B. Non-contrast–enhanced CT

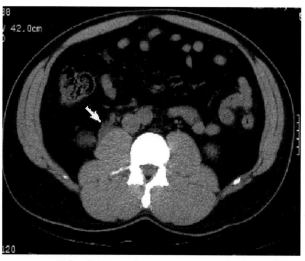

FIG. 87C. Non-contrast–enhanced CT

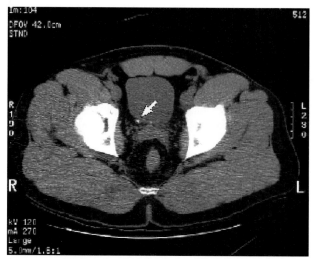

FIG. 87D. Non-contrast–enhanced CT

History

Right flank pain. Rule out ureteral calculus.

Findings

Figures 87A–D are non-contrast-enhanced spiral CT scans of the upper abdomen and pelvis. Note in Figures 87A–C the perirenal fluid (arrow) from forniceal rupture. In Figure 87D a distal ureteral calculus is identified at the level of the right ureterovesical junction (arrow).

Diagnosis

Distal right ureteral calculus.

Discussion

One advantage of CT when compared to urography and sonography, is its ability to identify subtle perirenal fluid collections from forniceal rupture caused by acute ureteral obstruction. Fluid may collect in a spoke-wheel fashion, dissecting between the fibrous lamellae of the perirenal space and along the proximal ureter. In the absence of infection, forniceal rupture is of little clinical concern, since fluid is quickly resorbed by abundant perirenal lymphatics.

References

Levin E. Acute renal and urinary tract disease. *Radiol Clin North Am* 1994; 32:989–1004.
Smith RC, Rosenfield AT, Choe KA, et al. Acute flank pain: comparison of non-contrast-enhanced CT and intravenous urography. *Radiology* 1995; 194:789–794.

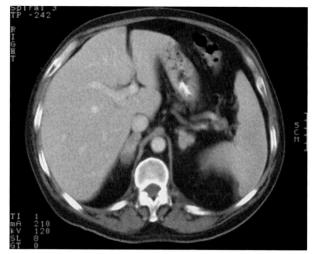

FIG. 91A. Contrast-enhanced CT

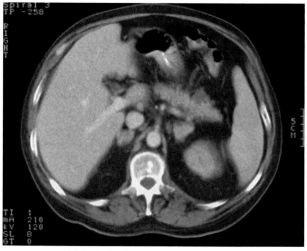

FIG. 91B. Contrast-enhanced CT

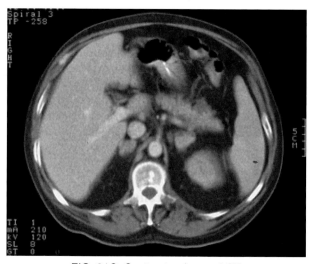

FIG. 91C. Contrast-enhanced CT

History

A 57-year-old male with known histoplasmosis and a recent onset of Addisons disease. A spiral CT scan was obtained to determine the extent of disease.

Findings

Spiral CT demonstrates enlargement of both adrenal glands, although they tend to maintain their triangular shape. There is no evidence of hemorrhage into either adrenal gland. No evidence of adenopathy or hepatosplenomegaly is noted.

Diagnosis

Disseminated histoplasmosis involving both adrenal gland.

Discussion

Spiral CT can rapidly evaluate the adrenal glands, especially if thin-section CT scans are employed. The differential diagnosis for bilaterally enlarged adrenal glands is extensive and ranges from hyperplasia or adenoma to metastatic disease or pheochromocytoma. In the present case, both adrenal glands are enlarged but tend to maintain an adrenal-type shape. There is no evidence of calcification or hemorrhage into either adrenal gland. One not uncommon cause of adrenal insufficiency or Addison disease is adrenal hemorrhage, often caused by anticoagulant therapy.

With the spread of acquired immune deficiency syndrome (AIDS), there has been an increased incidence of disseminated histoplasmosis, which was the case in this patient. Interestingly, this patient did not have AIDS. In the AIDS patient, disseminated histoplasmosis can occur by itself or as part of the spectrum of diseases accompanying the syndrome, including other infections or tumors such as Kaposi sarcoma.

Radin evaluated a series of abdominal CT scans in 16 patients with disseminated histoplasmosis. He found hepatomegaly in 63% of cases, splenomegaly in 38%, diffuse splenic hypoattenuation in 90%, bilateral adrenal enlargement or hypoattenuating masses in 13%, and enlarged lymph nodes in 44%.

The CT appearance of adrenal involvement by histoplasmosis is typically that of bilaterally enlarged glands. Interestingly, in one case of adrenal enlargement illustrated in Radin's article, both adrenal glands were enlarged but tended to maintain their adrenal-type shape. Adrenal enlargement due to histoplasmosis can occur in patients with disseminated histoplasmosis even without AIDS or AIDS-related complex. The importance of suggesting an inflammatory etiology is to avoid confusing the process with a malignancy, and to limit the extent of the patient's clinical and radiologic evaluation.

References

Davies SF. Histoplasmosis: update 1989. *Semin Respir Infect* 1990; 5:93–104.
Radin DR. Disseminated histoplasmosis: abdominal CT findings in 16 patients. *AJR* 1991; 157:955–958.
Wilson DA, Muchmore HG, Tisdal RG, Fahmy A, Pitha JV. Histoplasmosis of the adrenal glands studied by CT. *Radiology* 1984; 150:779–783.

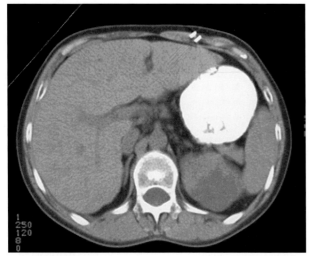

FIG. 92A. Non-contrast–enhanced CT

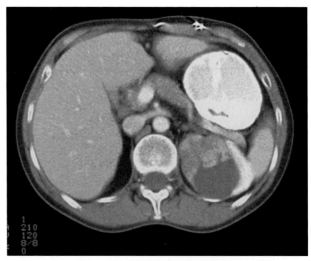

FIG. 92B. Contrast-enhanced CT

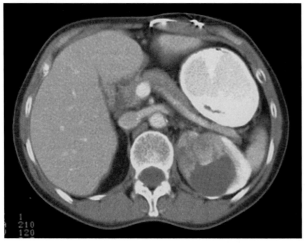

FIG. 92C. Contrast-enhanced CT

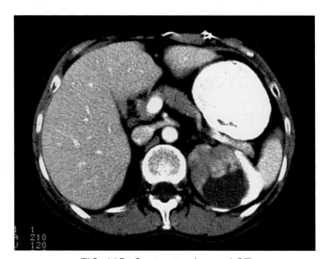

FIG. 92D. Contrast-enhanced CT

History

A 48-year-old female with a history of rheumatic heart disease and St. Jude replacements of her aortic and mitral valves. The patient was involved in an automobile accident, for which a CT scan was done and a mass was suggested in the left kidney. Serial CT scans were obtained and were felt to show that the mass was possibly growing. A spiral CT scan was obtained to better define the extent of disease and help, if needed, with preoperative surgical planning.

Findings

A non-contrast-enhanced CT scan through the kidney was obtained (Figure 92A) and demonstrated a cystic mass in the midportion of the left kidney. A spiral CT (Figure 92B–D) with rapid injection of contrast material demonstrated a mass in the left kidney. The mass had cystic and solid components. No evidence of adenopathy was seen, and the renal vein was normal.

Diagnosis

Mesoblastic nephroma of the kidney.

Discussion

The mass in this case does not meet any of the criteria for a simple cyst, and consists of a solid renal mass with both cystic and solid components. The most likely diagnosis in reviewing the CT scan preoperatively would be that of incidental renal-cell carcinoma. With the increased use of CT and ultrasound, renal carcinomas are in fact not uncommonly found incidentally. With the increase use of spiral CT, smaller renal-cell carcinomas are in fact being detected earlier. In one series, nearly one-third of resected renal cancers were detected serendipitously.

Other possibilities than a renal cell carcinoma in the differential diagnosis in this case would be lymphoma or a metastatic lesion. A metastasis can have a similar appearance to a primary renal tumor, particularly if the primary site is a melanoma.

At surgery, the tumor in this case was found to be a mesoblastic nephroma. Mesoblastic nephroma is a rare, typically benign tumor that is typically discovered in infancy. It is the most common solid renal mass in the first few months of life, and in most cases is homogeneously solid. However, hemorrhage, necrosis, or cystic degeneration are not uncommon, and may produce multiple cystic spaces resulting in a multiloculated mass as seen on CT. Hartman notes that most mesoblastic nephromas are detected in the first month of life and have to be differentiated from a multicystic kidney. One differential point in the younger patient is that the multicystic kidney (which is the most common source of a renal mass in the neonate) typically involves the entire kidney, while a mesoblastic nephroma involves a portion of the kidney. Mesoblastic nephromas are rarely ever found in the adult patient. Because they are usually considered to be benign tumors, no further evaluation or treatment is necessary.

Argons et al. note that mesoblastic nephroma is composed of spindle cells that grow by infiltration, using the preexisting nephromas as a scaffold. They authors note that mesoblastic nephromas are for the most part benign tumors, but that a subgroup is potentially more aggressive, with metastatic behavior having been documented. These cases tend to contain cystic areas of hemorrhage and necrosis, and Argons et al. note that these areas most commonly will resemble a cystic renal tumor.

The present examination shows images from the cortical medullary phase of CT image acquisition. A recent article suggests that this phase may potentially miss renal tumors that are very vascular or small, particularly if they are in the medullary zone. This may be true, but has not been a significant problem in our experience. However, in select cases, delayed scans or delayed image acquisition may be helpful.

References

Argons GA, Wagner BJ, Davidson AJ, Suarez ES. Multilocular cystic renal tumor in children: radiologic-pathologic correlation. *RadioGraphics* 1995; 15:653–669.

Cohen RH, Sherman LS, Korobkin M, Bass JC, Francis IR. Renal masses: assessment of corticomedullary-phase and nephrographic-phase CT scans. *Radiology* 1995; 196:445–451.

Hartman DS, Davis CJ, Sanders RC, Johns TT, Smirniotopoulos J, Goldman SM. The multiloculated renal mass: considerations and differential features. *RadioGraphics* 1987; 7:29–52.

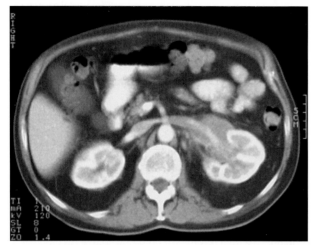

FIG. 93A. Contrast-enhanced CT

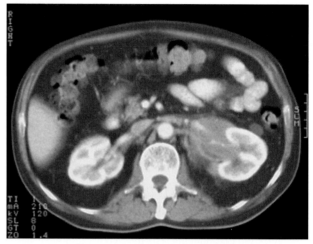

FIG. 93B. Contrast-enhanced CT

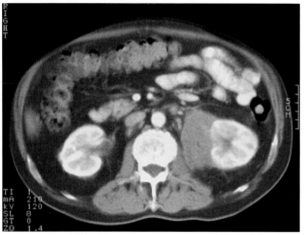

FIG. 93C. Contrast-enhanced CT

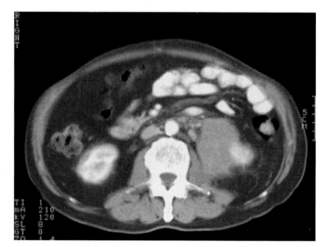

FIG. 93D. Contrast-enhanced CT

History

A 72-year-old male with a history of indolent follicular mixed lymphoma, stage IIIA, diagnosed 3 years earlier. He presented with abdominal pain and a metastatic lesion in the sternum. A CT scan was requested for evaluation of extent of disease.

Findings

A spiral CT scan of the abdomen demonstrates an infiltrating soft-tissue mass involving the left renal pelvis and perihilar zone. The renal artery and vein appear to extend through this infiltrating, homogeneous tumor mass. Differential diagnosis includes recurrent lymphoma as well as the possibility of other malignant tumors. A transitional-cell carcinoma of the renal pelvis is considered, although the pattern of extension seen in this case would be unusual with such a tumor. Also, if this lesion were a transitional cell carcinoma, the clear cortical medullary differentiation seen on the spiral CT scan would not be noted. This is more likely to be seen in lymphoma, which is more of a soft, infiltrative-type process.

Diagnosis

Mixed follicular-cell lymphoma.

Discussion

Spiral CT is an excellent means of staging lymphoma because of its ability to detect disease in nearly every organ and organ system in the abdominal cavity. The acquisition of data during the key vascular-enhancement phase appears to increase detection of disease in the liver and spleen, two organs that have always been difficult to evaluate with routine CT imaging in the patient with lymphoma.

The kidney is involved in up to one-third of cases of lymphoma according to autopsy series. The most common presentation of lymphoma is bilateral disease, and in the majority of cases is non-Hodgkin lymphoma. Renal involvement denotes stage IV Hodgkin disease.

The pattern of renal involvement by lymphoma is typically classified into four categories. The first is that of a solitary mass, which may or may not occur with associated paraaortic adenopathy. A second pattern is that of multiple masses with multiple nodules of varying size typically involving both kidneys. In most cases the kidneys are enlarged. The third pattern is diffuse infiltration of the kidney, in which the kidney on non-contrast-enhanced studies is enlarged and on contrast enhanced studies may show nephromegaly with either relatively normal enhancement, some decreased enhancement, or a persistent nephrograms. A fourth pattern is infiltration of the kidney by contiguous retroperitoneal disease. In this case the kidney is directly invaded or engulfed by adjacent tumor, with the renal outlines at times being very poorly defined. In select cases, lymphomatous infiltration of the perirenal space may also be seen.

In the present case, the fourth pattern is seen. The left kidney is infiltrated by disease extending into the renal pelvis. Interestingly, the kidneys appear to function normally, which is a hallmark of early direct extension by lymphoma. When obstruction is present, delayed function will be seen. The possibility of adenopathy extending into the kidney from a second source should be considered as well. However, our experience is that in most cases, adenopathy will not present as a smooth sheet of tumor as in the present case, but will typically show discrete masses, which may be individually outlined. In these cases, the most common type of involvement will be that of hydronephrosis. Lymphoma often tends to be a softer tumor and infiltrates the kidney.

References

Fishman EK, Kuhlman JE, Jones RJ. CT of lymphoma: spectrum of disease. *RadioGraphics* 1991; 11:647–669.

Hartman DS, Davis CJ Jr, Goldman SM, Friedman AC, Fritzsche P. Renal lymphoma: radiologic-pathologic correlation of 21 cases. *Radiology* 1992; 144:759–766.

Heiken JP, McClennan BL, Gold RP. Renal lymphoma. *Semin Ultrasound CT MR* 1986; 7(1):58–66.

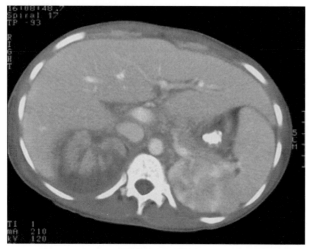

FIG. 94A. CT

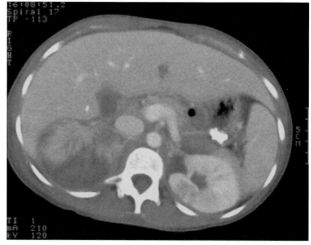

FIG. 94B. CT

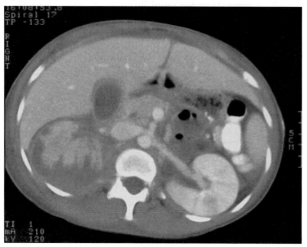

FIG. 94C. CT

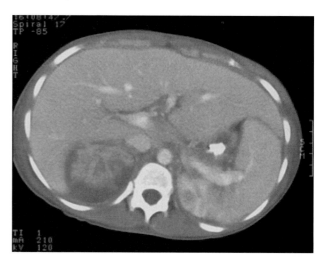

FIG. 94D. CT

History

A 23-year-old female developed persistent fevers following childbirth. Her urine was remarkable for a cloudy, white, particulate matter, and was sent for cultures. A CT scan was done for further evaluation.

Findings

A spiral CT scan demonstrates abnormal enhancement of the right kidney, with poor definition of a cortical medullary junction and irregular striations. A diffuse low-attenuation zone is present in the posterior portion of the right kidney. The renal vein appears normal. The differential diagnosis includes infection or infarction. The possibility of underlying renal tumor would be considered, but the appearance and clinical history in this case are not consistent with this diagnosis.

Diagnosis

Right renal pyelonephritis and abscess.

Discussion

Urine cultures in this patient grew *Escherichia coli*. Because of the extent of involvement on CT, it was felt that a percutaneous drainage of the kidney should be performed. A right renal tube was placed. The fluid from the tube drainage also was *E. coli*-positive. The patient was treated with trimethoprim/sulfamethoxazole and did well clinically, although subsequent CT scans documented a loss of cortex and decreased renal function.

In most patients with renal inflammatory disease the diagnosis is made either clinically or based on urine cultures, and radiologic imaging studies are not necessary. However, in some patients the clinical history is nonspecific and renal disease is only one of several clinical possibilities. In addition, in patients with known renal inflammatory disease who do not respond to a standard course of therapy, CT scanning may be done to look for complications such as abscess or extension of infection into the pararenal space.

With spiral CT, early-phase imaging detects changes in corticomedullary enhancement (40 to 50 seconds after injection), which is altered even with very mild inflammatory disease. In the present case the right kidney does not have normal renal enhancement because of an extensive inflammatory response. However, no evidence of extension into the peri- or pararenal space is noted. Although we recommend early-phase spiral imaging, delayed scans may also be helpful in defining the extent of inflammatory foci in the kidney.

The terminology for renal inflammatory disease has been somewhat confusing over the years, with many different terms used to represent the process seen in this case. Such terms include bacterial nephritis, lobar nephronia, or preabscess stage. A recent classification system has tried to simplify matters by using the terms "acute pyelonephritis" (unilateral vs. bilateral), "focal or multifocal vs. diffuse," and "with or without swelling." The present case would be best described as acute pyelonephritis, diffuse in nature, with swelling.

An interesting aspect of this case is the fact that the patient had recently given birth. Postpartum patients will not uncommonly have renal disease such as acute pyelonephritis. Although most patients with persistent fever are treated medically without imaging, a CT scan is valuable in select cases.

References

Rabushka LS, Fishman EK, Goldman SM. Pictorial review: computed tomography of renal inflammatory disease. *Urology* 1994; 44:473–480.

Soulen MC, Fishman EK, Goldman SM, Gatewood OM. Bacterial renal infection: role of CT. *Radiology* 1989; 172:703–707.

Talner L, Davidson A, Lebowitz R, Dalla Palma L, Goldman SM. Acute pyelonephritis: can we agree on terminology? *Radiology* 1994; 192:297–305.

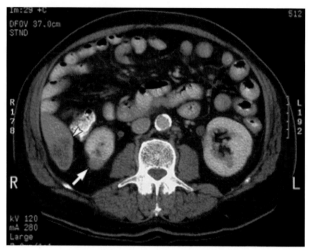

FIG. 95A. Contrast-enhanced CT

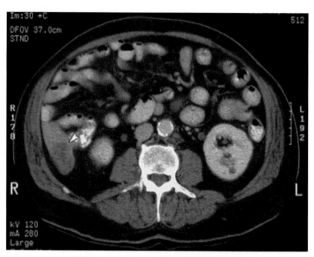

FIG. 95B. Contrast-enhanced CT

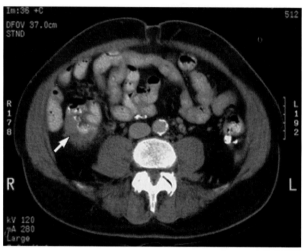

FIG. 95C. Contrast-enhanced CT

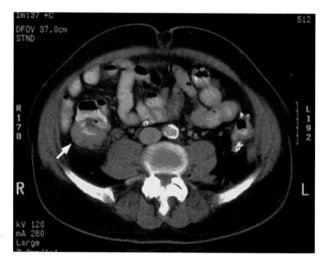

FIG. 95D. Contrast-enhanced CT

History

A 65-year-old male with vague right flank pain and fatigue.

Findings

Figures 95A–D are contrast-enhanced spiral CT scans of the abdomen. Note in Figure 95A an incidental, small, renal-cell carcinoma (arrow) extending from the lower pole of the right kidney. A focal hepatic lesion is identified in the poste-rior segment of the right lobe (arrowhe... D demonstrate marked mural thickening o... sistent with a cecal carcinoma (arrow).

Diagnosis

Cecal carcinoma metastatic to the liver; incidental renal-cell carcinoma.

Discussion

Two clinically unsuspected neoplasms were detected with CT in this patient: renal-cell carcinoma and cecal carcinoma. Renal neoplasms are the most commonly encountered inci-dental tumors identified with CT. Improved contrast-medium delivery with spiral CT, and lack of misregistration artifacts, provide increased sensitivity for incidental findings such as small renal and bowel neoplasms. The patient's fatigue was due to microcystic anemia caused by chronic blood loss from the colon cancer.

References

Bosniak MA. The small (less than or equal to 3.0 cm) renal parenchy-mal tumor: detection, diagnosis, and controversies. *Radiology* 1991; 179:307–317.

Curry NS. Small renal masses (lesions smaller than 3 cm): imaging evaluation and management. *AJR* 1995; 164:355–362.

McClennan BL. Oncologic imaging. Staging and follow-up of renal and adrenal carcinoma. *Cancer* 1991; 67:1199–1208.

Tsukamoto T, Kumamota Y, Yamazaki K, et al. Clinical analysis of incidentally found renal cell carcinomas. *Eur Urol* 1991; 19:109–113.

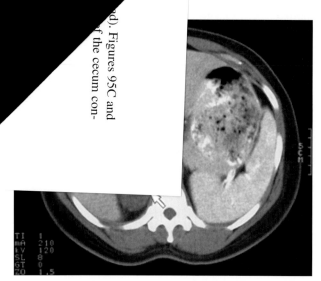

FIG. 96A. Contrast-enhanced CT

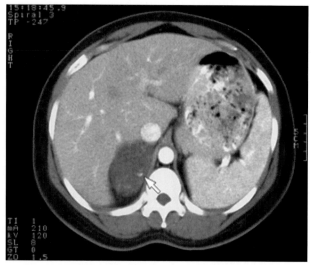

FIG. 96B. Contrast-enhanced CT

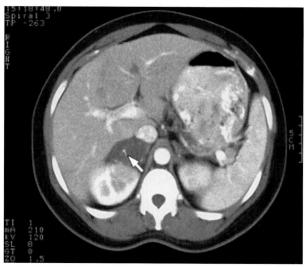

FIG. 96C. Contrast-enhanced CT

History

A 45-year-old female with a history of flank pain. An ultrasound study demonstrated a left adnexal mass and a right adrenal mass. A CT was ordered to evaluate the adrenal mass.

Findings

A spiral CT scan demonstrates a right adrenal mass approximately 5 cm in size. The mass is of low CT attenuation, with areas of septations and calcification (arrow). The left adrenal gland appears normal.

Diagnosis

Lymphangioma of the right adrenal gland.

Discussion

Spiral CT scanning is an excellent study for evaluation of the adrenal glands. In cases in which subtle lesions such as aldosteronomas are suspected, narrow collimation with small interscan gaps can be used and will help detect small lesions. In other cases, such as the one presented here, the appearance of the lesion becomes critical. This lesion is of low CT attenuation, measuring near fat density. At first glance this could be an adenoma, which commonly measures around –10 to +10 Hounsfield units (HU). However, this lesion does have foci of calcification, which would be unusual for adenoma. Also, the lesion is above the upper limits of size for which lesions can be described as incidental adenomas.

The possibility that this could represent a primary adrenal carcinoma or metastatic disease is considered. Adrenal carcinomas are usually of higher attenuation (50 to 70 HU), may enhance, and are not uncommonly calcified. Metastatic lesions to the adrenal gland are more common but rarely calcify. Also, except for melanoma, it is rare for lesions to be of low attenuation, and the appearance would therefore make the lesion in this case unlikely to be a metastatic or primary malignant tumor.

An uncommon benign tumor of the adrenal gland is a myelolipoma, which can be composed of various amounts of fat and myeloid tissue. These lesions contain calcification, but typically have areas within them that measure in the range of –100 HU. This could, however, be an atypical myolipoma. One final consideration would be that of hematoma of the adrenal gland. Chronic hematomas can be of low CT attenuation and may have calcification, although it would typically be in the wall of the lesion.

The lesion was removed and was a lymphangioma.

Lymphangiomas are rare tumors of the adrenal gland, and are benign lesions without any malignant potential.

References

Bernardino ME. Management of the asymptomatic patient with a unilateral adrenal mass. *Radiology* 1988; 166:121–123.

Casey LR, Cohen AJ, Wile AG, Dietrich RB. Giant adrenal myelolipomas: CT and MRI findings. *Abdom Imag* 1994; 19:165–167.

van Erkel AR, van Gils APG, Lequin M, Kruitwagen C, Bloem JL, Falke THM. CT and MR distinction of adenomas and nonadenomas of the adrenal gland. *J Comput Assist Tomogr* 1994; 18:432–438.

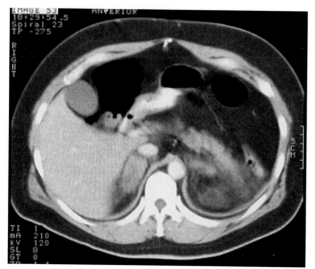

FIG. 97A. CT

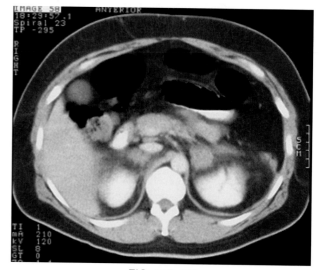

FIG. 97B. CT

History

A 45-year-old male with a history of Hodgkin disease and recent Trousseau syndrome. The patient developed acute abdominal and back pain, increasing over 24 hours. A CT scan was ordered with the clinical suspicion being acute pancreatitis.

Findings

A spiral CT scan demonstrates bilaterally enlarged adrenal glands, which appear to be of high CT attenuation, with some inflammation around the glands and extending toward the pararenal spaces.

Diagnosis

Acute bilateral adrenal hemorrhage secondary to anticoagulant therapy.

Discussion

The current role of anticoagulant therapy, whether for pulmonary embolism, venous thrombosis, or a patient at high risk for thromboembolic disease, is based on disease prevention and limiting disease progression. Anticoagulation can result in a variety of complications leading to increased patient morbidity and mortality. In many cases, the clinical presentation of these complications may be overlooked or confused with other pathologic processes. Spiral CT is commonly used for the evaluation of abdominal pain in the immunosuppressed patient. Spiral CT provides an examination that can be done rapidly while covering the entire abdomen. Because patients who are immunosuppressed can develop a wide range of complications, whether hematologic or infectious, spiral CT appears to be an excellent imaging strategy.

The clinical presentation of adrenal hemorrhage can be either occult, with the patient having Addison disease, or acute, with a hypertensive crisis, as in the patient presenting with an acute adrenal hemorrhage.

The classic CT appearance of adrenal hemorrhage is of adrenal glands that appear hyperdense relative to muscle and typically circular or oval in appearance. The typical size of the glands is approximately 3 to 5 cm. Hemorrhage may be unilateral or bilateral, but if bilateral may lead to acute adrenal insufficiency. Follow-up CT scans will typically show improvement in the disease process, with a decrease in size of the glands as well as in density. Calcification of the adrenal glands, either in the periphery or diffusely, may be one of the sequelae of prior adrenal hemorrhage. It is important to recognize adrenal hemorrhage, since the patient may otherwise be mismanaged, which can result in a life-threatening crisis. As in this case, adrenal hemorrhage is often not a clinical consideration, but the CT scan allows the radiologist to make the correct diagnosis.

Although it might seem logical that both the patient and treating physician are aware of the potential effects of anticoagulant medication, this is often not the case. Our experience has been that only in retrospect was the correct diagnosis obvious in a case of complication caused by such medication. In this case presentation, it was only retrospectively recognized that the patient had an elevated partial thromboplastin time (PTT).

References

Launbjerg J, Egeblad H, Heaf J, et al. Bleeding complications to oral anticoagulant therapy: multivariate analysis of 1010 treatment years in 551 outpatients. *J Intern Med* 1991; 229:351–355.

Levine MN, Hirsh J, Landefeld S, Raskob G. Hemorrhagic complications of anticoagulant treatment. *Chest* 1992; 102(4):352S–363S.

Scott WW, Fishman EK, Siegelman SS. Evaluation of abdominal pain in anticoagulated patients: the role of CT. *JAMA* 1984; 252:2053–2056.

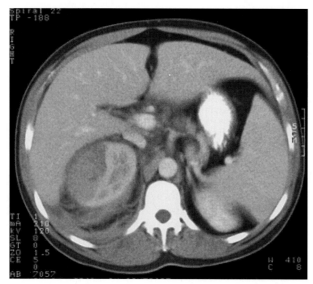

FIG. 98A. Contrast-enhanced CT

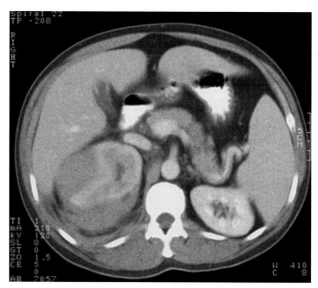

FIG. 98B. Contrast-enhanced CT

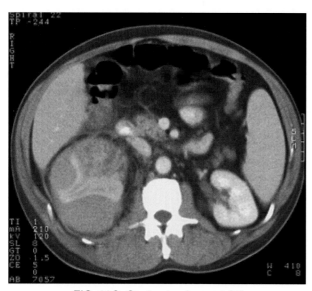

FIG. 98C. Contrast-enhanced CT

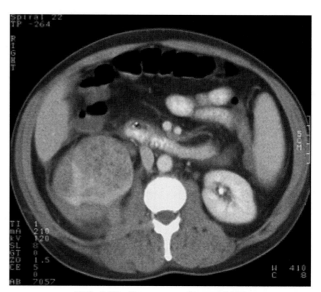

FIG. 98D. Contrast-enhanced CT

History

A 43-year-old white male with a history of acquired immune deficiency syndrome (AIDS). The patient presented with fever and abdominal pain localized to the right flank. He also has a history of Christmas disease, and had several recent episodes of hematuria. A CT scan was done to help determine the source of the flank pain and hematuria.

Findings

A spiral CT scan demonstrates normal enhancement of the left kidney. The right kidney shows irregular enhancement with some mass effect and high-density fluid (blood) in the perirenal and pararenal spaces. On scans through the upper portion of the kidney, a normal although compressed kidney was seen.

Diagnosis

Spontaneous perinephric and subcapsular renal hemorrhage.

Discussion

Spontaneous renal hemorrhage into the perinephric and/or subcapsular space is often an indirect sign of underlying primary renal pathology. Potential causes include tumors such as renal-cell carcinoma and angiomyolipoma, vascular processes such as arteriovenous (AV) malformations or polyarteritis nodosa, or underlying bleeding disorders such as hemophilia (or other bleeding disorders) and bleeding from anticoagulant therapy. CT scan clearly detect the presence and extent of bleeding, and in most cases reveal its cause.

Belville et al. reviewed a series of 18 consecutive patients with perinephric and subcapsular renal hemorrhage, and in 78% were able to make the correct diagnosis of the etiology of bleeding. The key CT finding was typically an underlying mass that was clearly distinct from the bleeding. A careful search for fat within the tumor was critical in making the diagnosis of a renal angiomyolipoma.

Spiral CT should be especially valuable in this potentially difficult group of patients. A set of scans obtained during the corticomedullary phase (40 to 50 seconds after initiation of injection) is ideal for detecting sites of bleeding, especially aneurysms, pseudoaneurysms, or AV malformations. Underlying vascular tumors should also be well defined at this time. A set of delayed scans may be useful for defining subtle tumors as well as in distinguishing a renal neoplasm from an abscess. Non-contrast-enhanced CT scans will show the extent of a renal hemorrhage but will be unlikely to add additional information the underlying cause of the bleeding.

In the case presented here, the clinical history of an underlying bleeding disorder like Christmas disease makes the likely cause of the perirenal hemorrhage a bit more obvious. What is especially interesting and well documented on the spiral CT scan is the extent of compression and distortion of the renal cortex caused by the extensive subcapsular component of the hemorrhage.

References

Belville JS, Morgantaler A, Loughlin KR, Tumeh SS. Spontaneous perinephric and subcapsular renal hemorrhage: evaluation with CT, US, and angiography. *Radiology* 1989; 172:733–738.

Kendall AR, Senay BA, Coll ME. Sponstaneous subcapsular renal hematoma: diagnosis and management. *J Urol* 1988; 139:246–250.

Schaner EG, Balow JE, Doppman JL. Computed tomography in the diagnosis of subcapsular and perirenal hematoma. *AJR* 1977; 129:83–88.

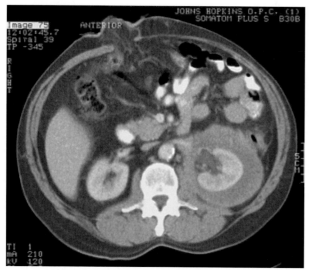

FIG. 99A. Axial scan

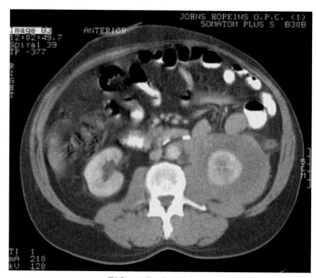

FIG. 99B. Axial scan

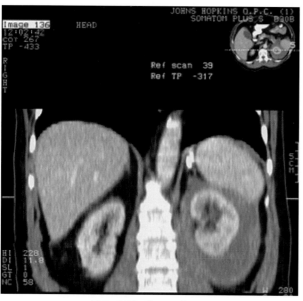

FIG. 99C. Coronal scan

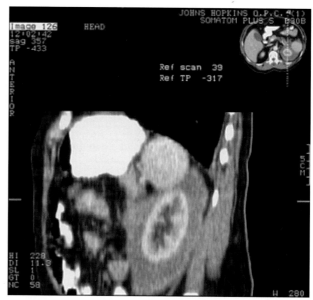

FIG. 99D. Sagittal scan

History

A 64-year-old male with a history of left flank pain.

Findings

A spiral CT scan demonstrates a large soft-tissue mass displacing and encasing the left kidney. The mass is of solid CT attenuation, appears to infiltrate the left perirenal space, and extends to and involves the left pararenal space posteriorly.

Diagnosis

Non-Hodgkin lymphoma involving the left kidney and perirenal and pararenal spaces.

Discussion

Lymphomatous involvement of the adrenal gland is most commonly a bilateral process involving single or multiple unilateral or bilateral renal masses. Direct extension into the kidney via a trans-sinus route can also occur. Probably the least common presentation is infiltration of the pararenal space, as in this case. The involvement of the kidney in non-Hodgkin lymphoma represents stage IV disease.

The present study also demonstrates the value of multiplanar reconstruction from spiral CT data. On the transaxial view there is clear definition of the extent of disease, with involvement of the perirenal space and apparent involvement of the pararenal space as well. Extension toward the left psoas muscle is also seen. The encasement and engulfment of the kidney is best appreciated, however, when looking at the coronal and sagittal views. Although in this case 8-mm-thick sections were obtained and reconstructed at 4-mm intervals, the lack of interscan breathing artifact on spiral CT makes the reconstruction of good quality. Obviously, if detailed analysis of vascular structures is needed from a multiplanar reconstruction, narrow interscan spacing and collimation are mandatory.

Ibukuro et al. showed that spiral CT angiography with multiplanar reformation has the potential in many cases to display vascular information similar to that provided by angiography, and in select cases to potentially replace angiography. However, Ibukuro et al. do note the importance of careful attention to technique for both data acquisition and data display.

References

Hartman DS, David CJ Jr, Goldman SM, Friedman AC, Fritzsche P. Renal lymphoma: radiologic-pathologic correlation of 21 cases. *Radiology* 1982; 144:759–766.

Ibukuro K, Charnsangavej C, Chasen MH, et al. Helical CT angiography with multiplanar reformation: techniques and clinical applications. *RadioGraphics* 1995; 15:671–682.

Jafri SZH, Bree RL, Amendola MA, et al. CT of renal and perirenal non-Hodgkin lymphoma. *AJR* 1982; 138:1101–1105.

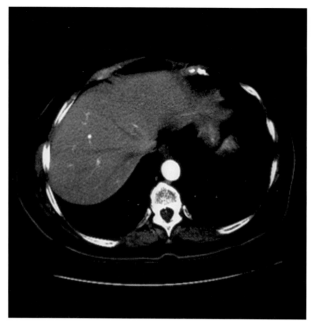

FIG. 100A. CT:arterial phase

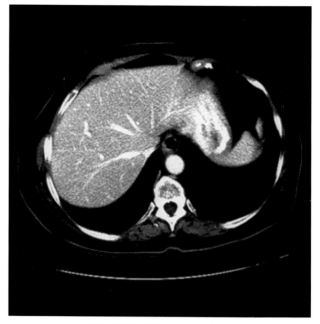

FIG. 100B. CT:venous phase

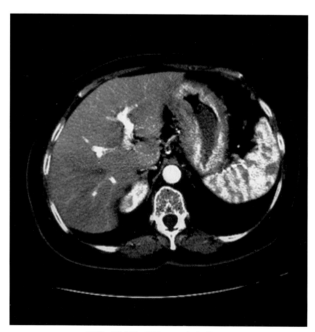

FIG. 100C. CT:arterial phase

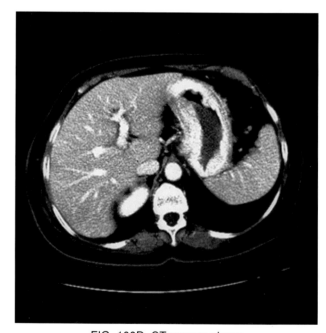

FIG. 100D. CT:venous phase

History

A 69-year-old female with suspected metastatic carcinoid tumor.

Findings

Figures 100A–D are arterial- and venous-phase scans obtained during a biphasic spiral CT of the liver. The liver is normal in attenuation throughout. Note in Figure 100A (obtained during the early arterial phase) the lack of enhancement of the hepatic veins. The hepatic veins are well demonstrated as enhancing vessels on the portal venous scan (Figure 100B). Compare the different density of the spleen during the early arterial Figure 100C and late portal venous Figure 100D phases. The mottled enhancement of the spleen is due to differential diffusion of contrast medium between the red pulp and white pulp of the spleen. In Figure 100D the spleen demonstrates uniform enhancement.

Diagnosis

Normal biphasic spiral CT of the liver and spleen.

Discussion

When interpreting biphasic spiral CT scans of the liver, it is important not to misconstrue normal, non-contrast, enhancing hepatic veins as low-attenuation "filling defects" or low-density masses on arterial-phase images. The spleen normally demonstrates a mottled appearance during the early arterial phase. It is often difficult to identify true lesions during the arterial phase of the spleen scan because of the heterogeneous patterns of enhancement.

References

Bluemke DA, Fishman EK. Spiral CT of the liver. *AJR* 1993; 160:787–792.
Zeman RK, Fox SH, Silverman PM, et al. Helical (spiral) CT of the abdomen. *AJR* 1993; 160:719–725.

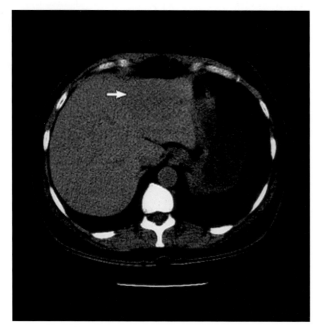

FIG. 101A. Non-contrast–enhanced CT

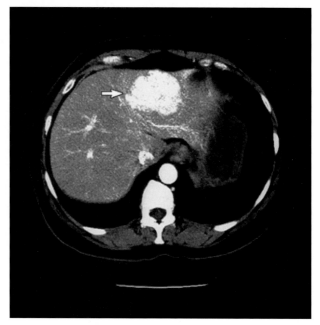

FIG. 101B. CT:arterial phase

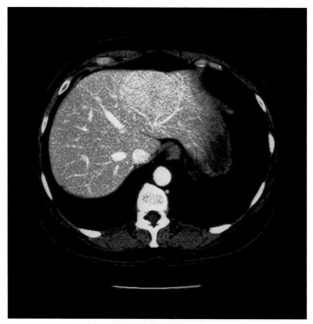

FIG. 101C. CT:venous phase

History

A 53-year-old female with an incidental liver mass discovered during routine gallbladder sonography. There is no known malignancy and no elevation of alpha fetoprotein.

Findings

Figure 101A is a non-contrast-enhanced scan of the liver demonstrating an ill-defined area of low attenuation in the lateral segment of the left lobe (arrow). Figure 101B is a scan obtained during the arterial phase of a biphasic spiral CT demonstrating a hypervascular lesion in the lateral segment of the left lobe (arrow). Figure 100C is a scan obtained during the portal-venous phase. The left-lobe lesion is nearly isoattenuating with the normal liver.

Diagnosis

Focal nodular hyperplasia.

Discussion

Focal nodular hyperplasia (FNH) is a benign hepatic lesion characterized pathologically by a central vascular scar containing and radiating fibrous septa. These lesions have been referred to as hepatic "hamartomas," because they contain normal hepatocytes and Kupffer cells. FNH is one of the few benign lesions of the liver that will appear hyperdense during the early arterial phase of a biphasic spiral CT scan. These lesions typically demonstrate intense enhancement during the arterial phase, with rapid washout of contrast. The liver is nearly isodense on both the non-contrast-enhanced scans and the late portal-venous scans. In 25% of patients a central scar can be identified on CT. Patients usually have normal liver function tests and no increase in α-fetoprotein. In selected patients, either magnetic resonance imaging (MRI) or technetium sulfur-colloid studies may help to confirm the diagnosis. There can, however, be overlap on MRI with hypervascular neoplasms such as fibrolamellar hepatocellular carcinoma, which may have a central scar. FNH does not have a capsule, unlike some forms of hepatocellular carcinoma. Occasionally, needle biopsy is required for definitive diagnosis.

References

Mathieu D, Rahmouni A, Anglade M-C, et al. Focal nodular hyperplasia of the liver: assessment with contrast-enhanced TurboFlash MR imaging. *Radiology* 1991; 180:25–30.
Ohtomo K, Itai Y, Yoshikawa K, et al. Hepatic tumors: dynamic MR imaging. *Radiology* 1987; 163:27–31.

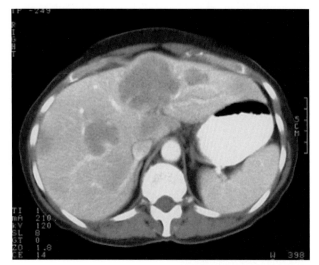

FIG. 102A. Contrast-enhanced CT

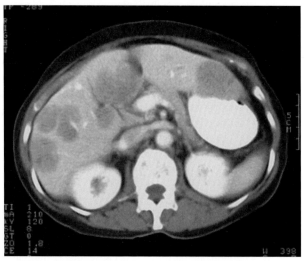

FIG. 102B. Contrast-enhanced CT

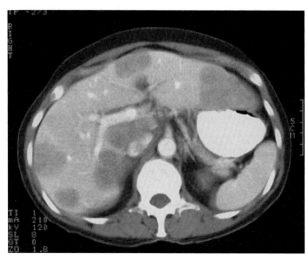

FIG. 102C. Contrast-enhanced CT

History

A 69-year-old female with B-cell lymphoma diagnosed several weeks earlier by lymph-node biopsy. CT was done for staging the extent of tissue.

Findings

A spiral CT scan demonstrates multiple, homogeneous, low-attenuation lesions in the liver. The liver is minimally enlarged. The lesions are generally hypovascular and show a minimal mass effect. No evidence of adenopathy is seen.

Diagnosis

Lymphoma of the liver.

Discussion

Infiltration of the liver is not uncommon in Hodgkin and non-Hodgkin lymphoma at the time of clinical presentation. Liver involvement is more common in patients with non-Hodgkin lymphoma (16%) than in patients with Hodgkin disease (10%). At autopsy, approximately 50% of patients with Hodgkin and non-Hodgkin lymphoma have hepatic involvement. In most cases, hepatic lymphoma is part of multiorgan involvement, and concurrent disease in the spleen, gastrointestinal tract, or lymph nodes is seen. In other cases, primary involvement of the liver may occur.

The CT appearance of lymphoma and the description in the pathologic literature are similar. Hodgkin disease is most commonly a diffuse infiltrating process, while non-Hodgkin disease may occur as either a diffuse infiltrating process or discrete tumor nodules. The ability of imaging studies to detect hepatic involvement by lymphoma has always been somewhat disappointing. This has been especially true in cases with nodules less than 1 cm in diameter or in cases with diffuse infiltration. A previous report by Zornoza and Ginaldi described a sensitivity of 57% and a specificity of 88% for conventional CT.

The CT appearance of lymphoma can be divided into three main categories: a solitary hepatic mass, multiple hepatic lesions, and diffuse infiltration. Based on these three categories it is easy to see how the CT appearance of lymphoma can simulate either primary hepatic tumors such as hepatoma or metastatic disease to the liver.

Detection of hepatic involvement by lymphoma should be enhanced with spiral CT. Optimization of contrast-medium delivery techniques, coupled with rapid volume-data acquisition, should help optimize lesion conspicuity. In the case presented, multiple hepatic lesions are seen as hypointense relative to normal liver, without a significant mass effect. This has been our experience with lymphoma.

We have not used biphasic spiral CT for evaluation of the liver in lymphoma, but it may be able to increase the success of lesion detection. Arterial-phase images may be especially valuable in detecting the infiltrating form of lymphoma and distinguishing it from parenchymal liver disease. However, to date no controlled study of the sensitivity and specificity of biphasic spiral CT has been done.

Primary hepatic lymphoma and secondary lymphomatous infiltration of the liver are being seen with increased incidence in patients with acquired immune deficiency syndrome (AIDS). In this group of immunocompromised patients, solid-organ involvement is more common than in other patient groups.

References

Bechtold RE, Karstaedt N, Wolfman NT, Glass TA. Prolonged hepatic enhancement on computed tomography in a case of hepatic lymphoma. *J Comput Assist Tomogr* 1985; 9:186–189.
Fishman EK, Kuhlman JE, Jones RJ. CT of lymphoma: spectrum of disease. *RadioGraphics* 1991; 11:647–669.
Zornoza J, Ginaldi S. Computed tomography in hepatic lymphoma. *Radiology* 1981; 138:405–410.

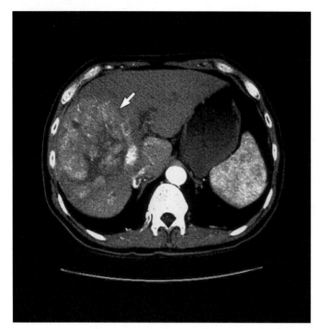

FIG. 103A. CT:arterial phase

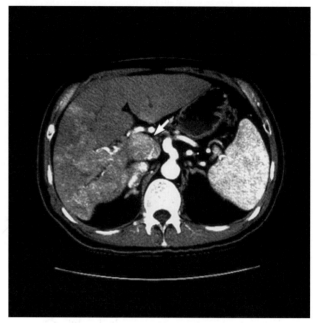

FIG. 103B. CT:arterial phase

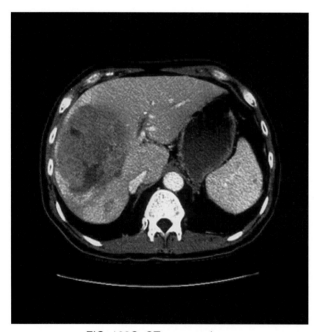

FIG. 103C. CT:venous phase

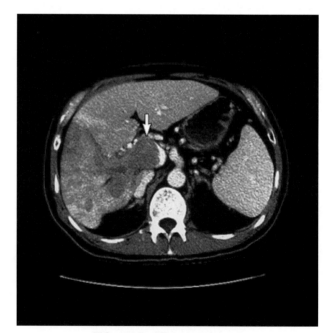

FIG. 103D. CT:venous phase

History

A 58-year-old male with elevated liver function test results and a longstanding history of hepatitis B.

Findings

Figures 103A and B are scans obtained during a rapid bolus dual-phase spiral CT study of the liver during the early arterial phase. Note a large enhancing lesion in the right lobe (arrow). Of particular note is that enhancing tumor thrombus is seen within the portal vein in Figure 103B (arrow). 103C and D are scans obtained during the portal venous demonstrating a low-density right-lobe mass with low-attenuation thrombus within the portal vein.

Diagnosis

Hepatocellular carcinoma with portal-venous invasion.

Discussion

Dual-phase spiral CT with a rapid bolus (5 ml/sec) is an excellent technique for the diagnosis of hepatocellular carcinoma. Early arterial-phase images obtained after a 25-second scan delay are particularly valuable in demonstrating small hypervascular satellite lesions and, as in this case, tumor invasion of the portal vein. Because isolated hepatocellular carcinomas are often treated surgically, the identification of multifocal disease is of critical importance to accurate staging of the disease. The demonstration of multifocal carcinoma often makes the patient unresectable for cure. The enhancement within the portal vein in the early arterial-phase images is diagnostic of tumor invasion of the portal vein. Scans obtained only during the portal-venous phase may demonstrate low-attenuation thrombus within the portal vein, which is not an uncommon finding in patients with cirrhosis. It may be difficult to accurately distinguish bland thrombus from tumor with portal-venous images alone.

Arterial-phase images improve the sensitivity for detection of hepatic hypervascular lesions such as hepatocellular carcinoma. Often these lesions are isodense during the equilibrium or portal venous phases and are only visualized during the early arterial portion of the spiral scan. There is a relatively short time interval in which to acquire predominantly arterial-phase images (approximately 25 to 55 seconds) from the start of the contrast injection. Thus, the ability to perform rapid back-to-back spiral scans is essential in order to accomplish dual-phase imaging of the liver. In patients with decreased cardiac output, there may be poor visualization of the liver during the arterial phase when a standard delay is used. These patients are probably best scanned with dynamic magnetic resonance imaging (MRI) using gadolinium and ultra-fast-gradient recalled images. Dual-phase spiral CT is limited by radiation and tube cooling. These factors are not applicable to MRI, because breath-hold sequences can be used over a long period of time in order to assure that there is adequate opacification of the arterial and portal-venous phases.

References

Bluemke DA, Urban BA, Fishman EK. Spiral CT of the liver: current applications. *Semin Ultrasound CT MR* 1994; 15:107–121.

Hollett MD, Jeffrey RB Jr, Nino-Murcia M, Jorgensen, MJ, Harris DP. Dual-phase helical CT of the liver: value of arterial phase scans in the detection of small (≤1.5 cm) malignant hepatic neoplasm. *AJR* 1995; 164:879–884.

Takayasu K, Moriyama N, Muramatsu U, et al. The diagnosis of small hepatocellular carcinomas: efficacy of various imaging procedures in 100 patients. *AJR* 1990; 155:49–54.

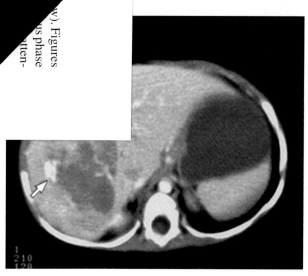

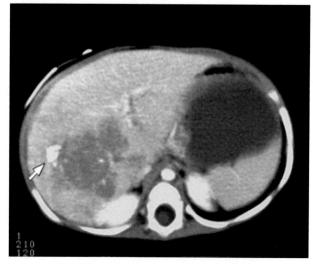

FIG. 104A. Contrast-enhanced CT

FIG. 104B. Contrast-enhanced CT

History

A 1-year-old male with failure to thrive and a palpable right abdominal mass.

Findings

A spiral CT scan demonstrates a large tumor infiltrating most of the right lobe of the liver, with coarse calcifications (arrow). The tumor appears to compress the inferior vena cava. The borders of the tumor are irregular and poorly defined.

Diagnosis

Hepatoblastoma.

Discussion

The classic liver tumors described in the pediatric patient are hepatoblastoma, hepatoma, and hemangioendothelioma. Hepatoblastoma is the most common symptomatic liver tumor in the patient under 5 years of age. Most cases present before age 3 and are more common in males than females. In a review of 50 cases of hepatoblastoma, Dachman et al. found that nearly all patients presented with hepatomegaly or a palpable mass.

The CT appearance of hepatoblastoma is that of a large mass (usually greater than 10 cm) which may be isolated to one lobe of the liver (usually the right lobe) or may be diffuse. The tumor has areas of calcification in more than 50% of cases, which could be described as coarse, stippled, or chunky in appearance. The tumors are usually hypervascular, and this is well demonstrated on a spiral CT scan. Lesions may have a hypervascular peripheral rims in select cases. Portal-vein invasion is not uncommon, especially in patients with infiltrating tumors.

Hepatoblastoma can usually be distinguished from hemangioendothelioma, because patients with the latter lesion usually present at an earlier age with symptoms such as congestive heart failure, and usually have a normal α-fetoprotein level. Hemangioendotheliomas are often multiple and may resemble hepatic hemangioma. Hepatoblastoma and hepatoma may look similar on CT, although hepatomas usually present at an older age and rarely (<5%) have hepatic calcification.

When planning therapy, key management decisions are based on tumor resectability. Spiral CT is most helpful in defining tumor extent and involvement of the hepatic and portal veins. Spiral CT with dual-phase liver imaging may be valuable in these patients for seeking arteriovenous (AV) shunting on arterial-phase images.

References

Dachman AH, Pakter RL, Ros PR, Fishman EK, Goodman ZD, Lichtenstein JE. Hepatoblastoma: radiologic-pathologic correlation in 50 cases. *Radiology* 1987; 164:15–19.

Gonzalez-Crussi F, Upton MP, Maurer HS. Hepatoblastoma: attempt at characterization of histologic subtypes. *Am J Surg Pathol* 1982; 6(7):599–612.

Korobkin MT, Kirks DR, Sullivan DC, Mills SR, Bowie JD. Computed tomography of primary liver tumors in children. *Radiology* 1091; 139:431–435.

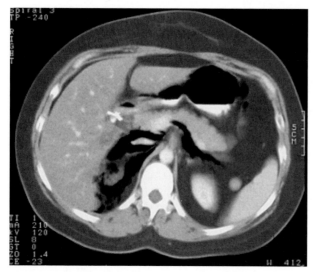

FIG. 105A. Contrast-enhanced CT

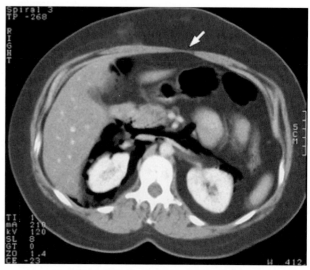

FIG. 105B. Contrast-enhanced CT

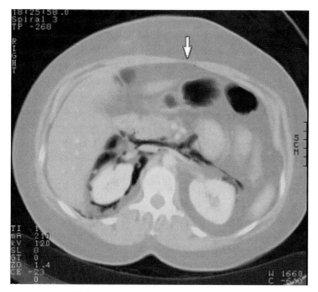

FIG. 105C. Contrast-enhanced CT

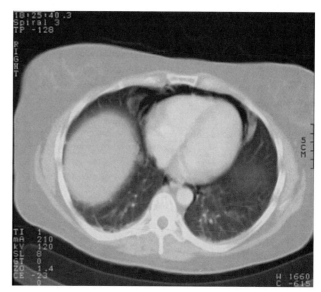

FIG. 105D. Contrast-enhanced CT

History

A 39-year-old female with a history of persistent right-upper-quadrant pain despite cholecystectomy. An Endoscopic Retrograde Cholangiopancreatography (ERCP) with sphincterotomy was done for further evaluation. Following the ERCP the patient developed increasing abdominal pain.

Findings

A spiral CT scan demonstrates free air in the retroperitoneum outlining the inferior vena cava, right kidney, and posterior portion of the pancreas. Air also dissected upward into the mediastinum and into the right lower quadrant around the colon. The patient was admitted and treated conservatively without further complication.

Diagnosis

Perforation of the duodenum as a complication of ERCP with sphincterotomy.

Discussion

This case is an excellent demonstration of the use of CT in the evaluation of iatrogenic complications, and of the ability to use the information generated for patient management. The patient underwent ERCP with sphincterotomy for possible bile-duct stones or papillary stenosis. One of the complications of ERCP with sphincterotomy is perforation. This complication can be noted during or immediately after the procedure. As in this case, the amount of air present can be extensive and a cause of great concern.

Complications of ERCP with sphincterotomy are reported in 2.5 to 11.7% of cases, with the severity of complications running the gamut from a mild asymptomatic increase in amylase levels to hemorrhagic pancreatitis, septic shock, and death. We previously reviewed a series of 36 patients referred for CT following ERCP with sphincterotomy for possible complications. Complications included acute pancreatitis (23 cases), duodenal perforation (11 cases), retroperitoneal dissection by air (4 cases), pneumoperitoneum (4 cases), and retroperitoneal abscess (2 cases). Eight patients had normal CT scans except for air and/or contrast medium in the biliary tree. Through the use of CT as a guide, 31 of 36 patients were successfully managed conservatively with antibiotics, intravenous-fluids, and restriction of oral intake. Four patients required surgical intervention.

In the present case, one of the helpful CT findings we noticed was that although there was extensive air in the retroperitoneum, there was essentially no inflammation. In cases requiring surgical intervention, extensive fluid or inflammation is usually present, commonly in the right pararenal space and dissecting down toward the right lower quadrant. This study also demonstrates how easily air in the abdomen can dissect into the chest.

References

Bilbao MK, Dotter CT, Lee TG, Katon RM. Complications of endoscopic retrograde cholangiopancreatography (ERCP). *Gastroenterology* 1976; 70:314–320.

Byrne P, Leung JWC, Cotton PB. Retroperitoneal perforation during duodenoscopic sphincterotomy. *Radiology* 1984; 150:383–384.

Kuhlman JE, Fishman EK, Milligan FD, Siegelman SS. Complications of endoscopic retrograde sphincterotomy: computed tomographic evaluation. *Gastrointest Radiol* 1989; 14:127–132.

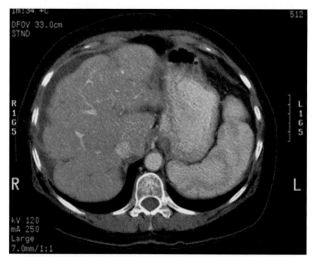

FIG. 106A. Contrast-enhanced CT

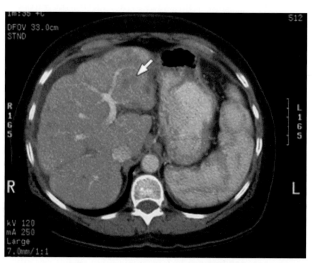

FIG. 106B. Contrast-enhanced CT

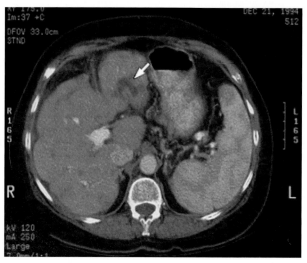

FIG. 106C. Contrast-enhanced CT

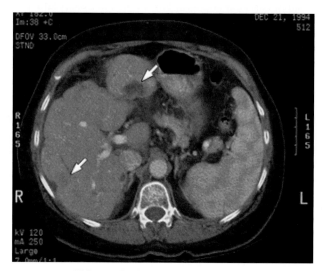

FIG. 106D. Contrast-enhanced CT

History

A 61-year-old female who had undergone three cycles of chemotherapy for metastatic carcinoma of the breast.

Findings

Figures 106A–D are spiral CT scans of the liver following contrast enhancement. Note on all four images the marked scarring of the surface of the liver and the surrounding ascites. Focal hepatic lesions are noted in the left lobe and posterior segment of the right lobe (arrows).

Diagnosis

Nodular regenerative hyperplasia of the liver following chemotherapy for metastatic carcinoma of the breast.

Discussion

The CT appearance of the liver in this patient mimics advanced cirrhosis because of the irregular liver contour, the surrounding ascites, and the moderate splenomegaly. This appearance has recently been described following chemotherapy for metastatic carcinoma of the breast. It is likely that the hepatotoxic effect of chemotherapy results in areas of atrophy and nodular regenerative hyperplasia. The focal low-density lesions may not represent residual tumor but areas of hepatic injury and fibrosis.

References

Shirkhoda A, Baird S. Morphologic changes of the liver following chemotherapy for metastatic breast carcinoma: CT findings. *Abdom Imag* 1994; 19:39–42.
Young ST, Paulson EK, Washington K, Gulliver DJ, Vredenburgh JJ, Baker ME. CT of the liver in patients with metastatic breast carcinoma treated by chemotherapy: findings simulating cirrhosis. *AJR* 1994; 153:1385–1388.

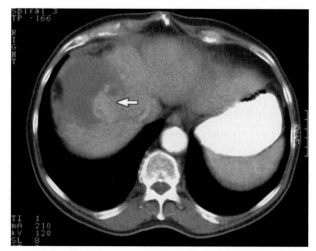

FIG. 107A. Contrast-enhanced CT

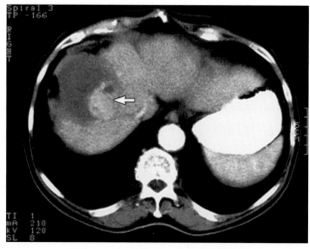

FIG. 107B. Contrast-enhanced CT

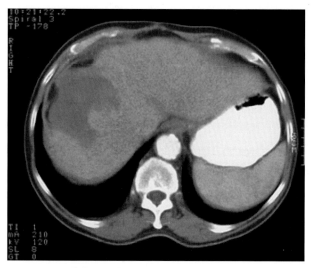

FIG. 107C. Contrast-enhanced CT

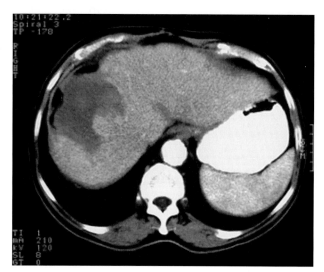

FIG. 107D. Contrast-enhanced CT

History

A 73-year-old male with a repeat CT scan 6 months after hepatic cryosurgery for hepatocellular carcinoma.

Findings

A spiral CT scan demonstrates a low-density lesson at the site of cryosurgery. There appear to be enhancing nodules (arrow) in the periphery of the cryolesion consistent with tumor recurrence.

Diagnosis

Recurrent hepatocellular carcinoma.

Discussion

Hepatic cryosurgery is a new treatment modality that offers the potential for curative treatment of both primary and metastatic tumors in the liver. Cryosurgery is typically used in the patient for whom classic hepatic resection is impossible because of tumor location, multiplicity of lesions, or the patient's poor overall condition.

The CT appearance of the liver following cryosurgery has recently been described. A series of 28 cryolesions were reviewed in 14 patients during periods 4 to 16 days following the procedure. Cryolesions were typically hypodense and extended to the liver capsule. Somewhat more than one third of the lesions contained air and over 90% contained areas of hemorrhage. Cryolesions were predominantly wedge-shaped (54%), rounded (29%), or tear-drop shaped (21%). In time, successful zones of cryosurgery may fill in or scar, so that the original site of cryosurgery is poorly defined. In the present case there appeared to be tumor nodules developing and increasing in size at the edge of the cryosurgery lesion. This represented tumor recurrence.

Other complications seen in the cryosurgery patient besides recurrence include hepatic abscesses, infarcts, or hemorrhage. The true effect of cryosurgery, in terms of long-term success or failure, is a subject of much interest. It may represent a new technique that could be performed percutaneously without an open surgical procedure. However, further investigation is necessary.

References

Gage AA, Fazekas G, Riley EE. Freezing injury to large blood vessels in dogs with comments on the effect of experimental freezing of bile ducts. *Surgery* 1967; 61:748–754.

Gage AM, Montes M, Gage AA. Destruction of hepatic and splenic tissue by freezing and heating. *Cryobiology* 1982; 19:172–179.

Kuszyk BS, Choti MA, Urban BA, Chambers TP, Bluemke DA, Stizmann JV, Fishman EK. Hepatic tumors treated by cryosurgery: normal CT appearance. *AJR* 199; 166:363–368.

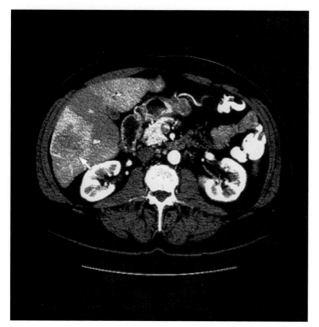

FIG. 108A. CT:arterial phase

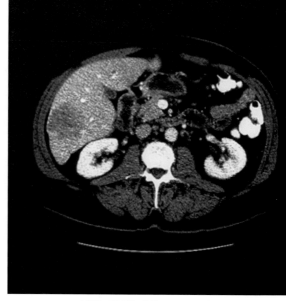

FIG. 108B. CT:venous phase

History

A 62-year-old male with known colon cancer and vague right-upper-quadrant pain. Rule out metastases.

Findings

Figure 108A is a scan obtained during the arterial phase of a biphasic spiral CT study of the liver. Note the hypodense lesion outlined by the intense peripheral rim of enhancement in the posterior segment of the right lobe (arrow). Figure 108B is a scan obtained during the portal venous phase, again demonstrating the lesion in the right lobe of the liver. The peripheral-rim enhancement is no longer evident.

Diagnosis

Colon cancer metastatic to the liver, with perilesional flow on arterial-phase images.

Discussion

Hepatic metastases demonstrate a variety of flow patterns on biphasic spiral CT. Central lesions that obstruct the portal veins may cause a compensatory increase in hepatic arterial flow to the segment involved by tumor. This may be evident only on arterial-phase images, because transiently increased hepatic attenuation may rapidly decrease during the portal-venous phase. Other lesions may demonstrate peripheral vascularity along the margin of the tumor, with a "peripheral halo" or ring pattern. In this patient the increased perilesional flow involved a larger segment than a peripheral ring of enhancement. This was probably due to portal venous obstruction with resultant increased flow in the hepatic artery in the posterior segment of the right lobe. It is important to recognize that this enhancing tissue is not viable tumor, but is due to flow phenomenon. In this patient the actual size of the tumor was better estimated on the portal-venous-phase images.

References

Bluemke DA, Fishman EK. Spiral CT of the liver. *AJR* 1993; 160:787–792.
Zeman RK, Fox SH, Silverman PM, et al. Helical (spiral) CT of the abdomen. *AJR* 1993; 160:719–725.

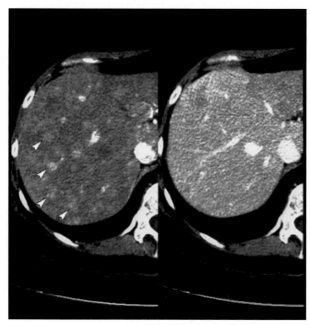

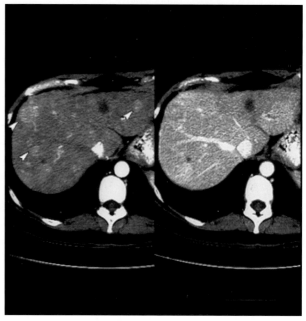

FIG. 109A. CT:arterial/venous phase

FIG. 109B. CT:arterial/venous phase

History

A 59-year-old patient with breast cancer. Rule out liver metastases.

Findings

Figures 109A and B are side-by-side comparisons of arterial and portal venous-phase scans of the liver obtained during a biphasic spiral CT examination. Note the multiple hyperattenuating foci on the arterial phase (arrowheads), which are difficult to identify in the portal-venous phase.

Diagnosis

Hepatic metastases from carcinoma of the breast.

Discussion

Dynamic contrast-enhanced CT of the liver for metastatic breast carcinoma has been notoriously inaccurate. This is due not only to the microscopic nature of the lesions, but to the fact that these metastases are often isodense when viewed on portal venous-phase images. Adenocarcinoma of the breast, when metastatic to the liver, has not been traditionally considered a "hypervascular" lesion. In some patients, however, metastases are hypervascular on early arterial-phase scans and are not apparent on portal-venous-phase images. Patients with suspected metastatic carcinoma of the breast should therefore be imaged with a rapid bolus, biphasic spiral CT technique. At autopsy, this patient's liver was virtually replaced by tumor, much of which was microscopic. However, many of the lesions clearly visualized on the arterial-phase images were not apparent on the portal-venous-phase images.

References

Caskey CI, Scataridge JC, Fishman EK, Distribution of metastases in breast carcinoma: CT evaluation of the abdomen. *Clin Imag* 1991; 15:166–171.

Hollett MD, Jeffrey RB Jr, Nino-Murcia M, Jorgensen, MJ, Harris DP. Dual-phase helical CT of the liver: value of arterial phase scans in the detection of small (≤1.5 cm) malignant hepatic neoplasms. *AJR* 1995; 164:879–884.

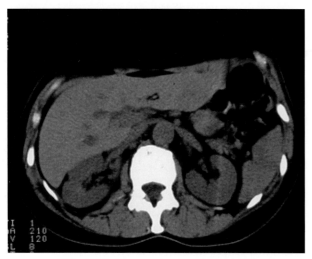

FIG. 110A. Non-contrast–enhanced CT

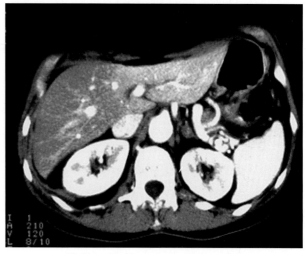

FIG. 110B. Contrast-enhanced CT

History

A 62-year-old female with a history of a poorly differentiated adenocarcinoma of the lung. The patient had been treated with chemotherapy and radiation therapy.

Findings

Non-contrast-enhanced CT scans of the liver demonstrate no evidence of metastatic liver disease. Spiral CT with contrast enhancement demonstrates differential enhancement of the liver, with the portion of the liver including the right lobe being of lower CT attenuation than the medial portion of the liver (Fig. 110B).

Diagnosis

Radiation-induced hepatic injury.

Discussion

Radiation injury to the liver can be a sequela of external-beam irradiation to a primary or metastatic tumor of the liver, or a result of hepatic injury when the liver is within the therapy field, such as in this patient with a right-lower-lung tumor. On non-contrast-enhanced CT, radiation injury is usually not detected, because the attenuation value of both normal and irradiated liver is equivalent. Following infusion of iodinated contrast medium there is typically an obvious difference in attenuation. The radiated field is defined by lower CT attenuation, and its boundaries are outlined by sharp margins corresponding to the therapy port.

We have seen several cases in which the irradiated liver is hyperdense on delayed scans (20 to 40 minutes after injection) relative to the normal, non-irradiated liver. This may be due to delayed excretion of contrast material or to increased pooling of such material in the injured hepatocytes. This appearance is most common about 2 months after therapy, and may resolve about 4 months later without any significant sequaele. Most patients with radiation injury have a radiation dose of more than 37 Gy.

Pathologically, radiation injury results in hyperemia, distended hepatic sinusoids, hepatic cell loss, and eventual fibrosis of small hepatic veins. Although in most cases the liver will appear normal on subsequent CT studies (after 6 months), in other cases focal fibrosis or atrophy may occur. Compensatory hypertrophy may also occur in non-irradiated portions of the liver.

The great majority of patients with CT changes reflecting hepatic radiation injury will be either asymptomatic or have minimally elevated liver function test results. The classic clinical triad of radiation hepatitis: abnormal liver function tests (elevated alkaline phosphatase only), nonmalignant ascites, and hepatomegaly, is uncommon. When it does occur, it is usually in patients who have had high-dose radiation therapy, and usually appears 2 to 6 weeks after the completion of therapy. The importance of the CT diagnosis of radiation injury to the liver is twofold. First is to not confuse such injury with hepatic tumor or metastatic disease. Second is in the patient with abnormal liver function and in whom tumor is a clinical consideration. In these cases CT can suggest the correct diagnosis and prevent a needless and expensive diagnostic workup.

With spiral CT the attenuation differences are clearly defined, although it is rare to see changes in vessel caliber in the liver. Another important feature that may be helpful with spiral CT is the lack of a mass effect in case of radiation injury to the liver. This diagnostic point could be helpful in cases of suspected or known tumor within the irradiated liver tissue.

References

Jeffrey RB Jr, Moss AA, Quivey JM, Federle MP, Wara WM. CT of radiation-induced hepatic injury. *AJR* 1980; 135:445–448.

Lawrence TS, Ten Haken RK, Kessler ML, et al. The use of 3D dose volume analysis to predict radiation hepatitis. *Int J Rad Oncol Biol Phys* 1992; 23:781–788.

Yamasaki SA, Marn CS, Francis IR, Robertson JM, Lawrence TS. High-dose localized radiation therapy for treatment of hepatic malignant tumors: CT findings and their relation to radiation hepatitis. *AJR* 1995; 165:79–84.

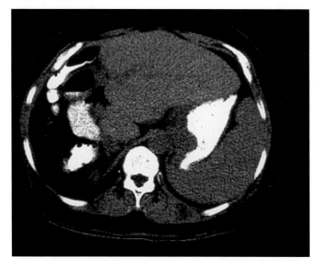

FIG. 111A. Non-contrast–enhanced CT

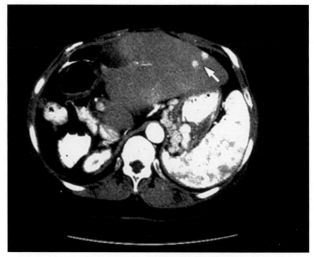

FIG. 111B. CT:arterial phase

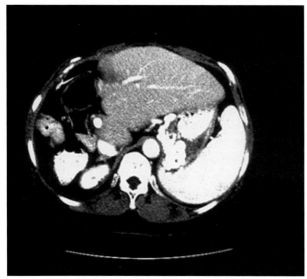

FIG. 111C. CT:venous phase

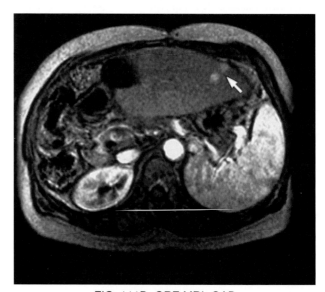

FIG. 111D. GRE MRI+GAD

History

A patient who underwent resection of a right-lobe hepatoma. The patient has a rising α-fetoprotein concentration.

Findings

Figure 111A is a non-contrast-enhanced scan of the liver demonstrating no focal abnormalities. Figure 111B is an arterial-phase image of a biphasic spiral CT study demonstrating two small enhancing tumor nodules in the lateral segment of the left lobe (arrow). Figure 111C is a scan obtained during the portal venous phase demonstrating no focal abnormalities. Figure 111D is a magnetic resonance imaging (MRI) scan immediately following an injection of gadolinium, using an ultrafast-gradient recalled sequence. Again, notice the enhancing tumor nodules in the lateral segment of the left lobe (arrow).

Diagnosis

Recurrent hepatocellular carcinoma seen only on arterial-phase images.

Discussion

This case nicely illustrates the value of arterial-phase images in diagnosing small hepatocellular carcinomas. The lesions were not visible on either the non-contrast-enhanced or portal-venous-phase scans. If a dynamic bolus CT scan had been performed, these lesions would have been missed because of the inability to obtain arterial-phase imaging. In patients who are not able to receive intravenous iodinated contrast medium, gadolinium-enhanced MRI can be of value in identifying hypervascular lesions, as in this case. For optimal lesion detection, immediate postinjection scans must be obtained in addition to scans at 1 to 3 minutes. One of the main advantages of MRI is that multiple acquisitions can be performed to characterize the temporal pattern of enhancement without radiation exposure.

References

Bluemke DA, Soyer P, Fishman EK. "Spiral CT evaluation of liver tumors." In: Fishman EK, Jeffrey RB Jr, (eds.): *Spiral CT: Principles, Techniques, and Clinical Applications*. New York: Raven Press, 1994, pp. 25–45.
Hollett MD, Jeffrey RB Jr, Nino-Murcia M, Jorgensen, MJ, Harris DP. Dual-phase helical CT of the liver: value of arterial phase scans in the detection of small (≤1.5 cm) malignant hepatic neoplasms. *AJR* 1995; 164:879–884.

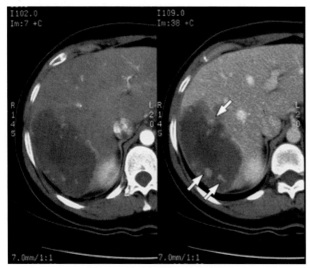

FIG. 112A. CT:arterial phase

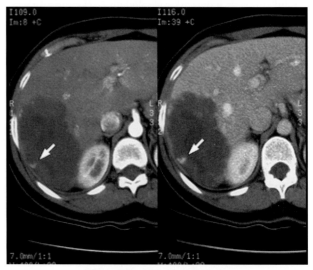

FIG. 112B. CT:arterial phase

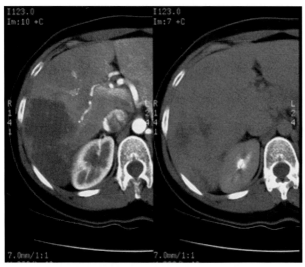

FIG. 112C. CT:arterial/venous phase

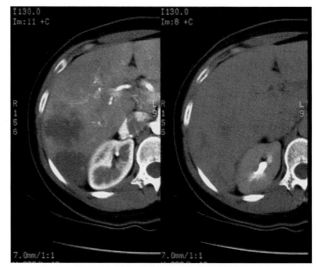

FIG. 112D. CT:arterial/venous phase

History

Incidental hepatic mass noted on a screening ultrasound examination.

Findings

Figures 112A and B are scans obtained during the arterial phase of a biphasic spiral CT study of the liver. Note the peripheral "puddling" of contrast medium at the margins of the lesion (arrow). The peripheral puddling is discontinuous and does not represent true "rim" enhancement. Figures 112C and D are side-by-side comparisons of arterial-and portal-venous-phase images demonstrating significant "filling in" of the lesion on the delayed portal venous images.

Diagnosis

Cavernous hemangioma of the liver demonstrated by biphasic spiral CT.

Discussion

Prior to the development of biphasic spiral CT, either tagged red-cell nuclear medicine scans or a single-station, dynamic CT scan was done to evaluate the liver for possible hemangioma. The disadvantage of the CT technique was that only a single area of the liver could be imaged. With biphasic spiral CT with breath-holding, however, the entire liver can be imaged twice with two separate breath-holds. The CT diagnosis of hemangioma rests almost entirely on the pattern of enhancement (i.e., identification of nodular peripheral puddling that is discontinuous). Rim enhancement suggests a malignant tumor or abscess. Many large cavernous hemangiomas will have central scarring or calcification and will not fill in completely. However, a diagnosis of hemangioma can be established when a characteristic pattern of "nodular puddling" is clearly identified by CT.

References

Ito K, Honjo K, Matsumoto T, et al. Distinction of hemangiomas from hepatic tumors with delayed enhancement by incremental dynamic CT. *J Comput Assist Tomogr* 1992; 16:572–577.

Quinn SF, Benjamin GG. Hepatic cavernous hemangiomas: simple diagnostic sign with dynamic bolus CT. *Radiology* 1992; 182:545–548.

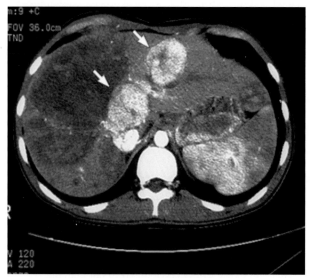

FIG. 113A. CT:arterial phase

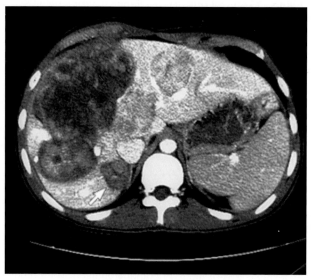

FIG. 113B. CT:venous phase

History

Cirrhosis with deteriorating liver function test valves. Rule out hepatocellular carcinoma.

Findings

Figure 113A is a scan obtained during the arterial phase of a biphasic spiral CT study of the liver. Note enhancing lesions in the caudate and left lobes (arrows). A large, low-attenuation lesion is seen laterally, involving the right lobe and the medial segment of the left lobe. Figure 113B is a scan obtained during the portal venous phase demonstrating better definition of the low-attenuation lesion in the right lobe and medial segment of the left lobe. In addition, a second low-attenuation lesion is seen immediately posterior to the intrahepatic inferior vena cava (arrow). The hypervascular lesions, previously quite conspicuous on the arterial phase, have diminished in density on the portal venous phase, and are nearly isoattenuating.

Diagnosis

Multifocal hepatocellular carcinoma.

Discussion

The right-lobe lesion in this patient was biopsied under ultrasound guidance. Cytology proved nondiagnostic, because only necrotic tissue and debris were recovered. This could have been predicted on the basis of the biphasic spiral CT because the lesion showed minimal enhancement on both arterial-and portal-venous-phase images, suggesting extensive necrosis. The lesions in the left lobe and in a caudate left lobe in this patient were identified more clearly during arterial-phase imaging. Tumor enhancement typically has a rounded or oval configuration. Arterial-phase enhancement is diagnostic of viable tumor. Because of rapid washout of contrast medium, the lesions may become isodense during the portal venous phase. Necrotic lesions, however, will almost always be best appreciated on the portal-venous images. A repeat biopsy of the left-lobe lesion was positive for hepatocellular carcinoma.

References

Hollett MD, Jeffrey RB Jr, Nino-Murcia M, Jorgensen, MJ, Harris DP. Dual-phase helical CT of the liver: value of arterial phase scans in the detection of small (≤1.5 cm) malignant hepatic neoplasms. *AJR* 1995; 164:879–884.
Patten RM, Byun JY, Freeny PC. CT of hypervascular hepatic tumors: are unenhanced scans necessary for diagnosis? *AJR* 1993; 161:979–984.

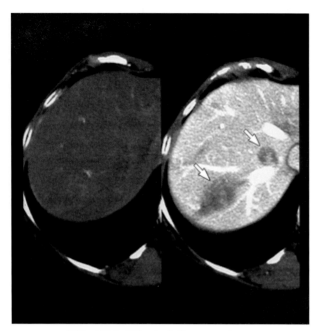

FIG. 116A. CT:arterial/venous phase

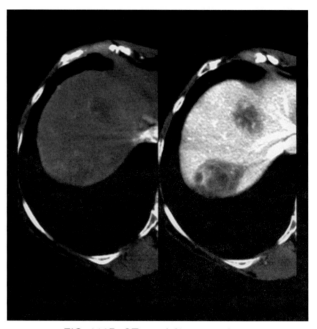

FIG. 116B. CT:arterial/venous phase

History

Carcinoid tumor of the small bowel. Rule out liver metastasis.

Findings

Figures 116A and B are side-by-side comparisons of arterial- and portal-venous-phase images from a biphasic spiral CT scan of the liver. Notice that the lesions are difficult to visualize on the arterial-phase images. The lesions are best identified during the portal venous phase (arrows), when there is significant enhancement of the hepatic parenchyma.

Diagnosis

Necrotic liver metastases from small-bowel carcinoid.

Discussion

Carcinoid and other neuroendocrine metastases are typically hypervascular lesions and often best visualized on arterial-phase images. With necrotic lesions, however, there is poor contrast enhancement during the early arterial phase. As is true with necrotic lesions in general, these abnormalities are best imaged during the portal venous phase. One of the advantages of the biphasic technique is that by combining both phases, some lesions that are hypervascular are best seen in the arterial phase, whereas necrotic lesions are better seen in the portal venous phase.

References

Bluemke DA, Soyer P, Fishman EK. "Spiral CT evaluation of liver tumors." In: Fishman EK, Jeffrey RB Jr, (eds.). *Spiral CT: Principles, Techniques, and Clinical Applications.* New York: Raven Press, 1994, pp. 25–45.

Hollett MD, Jeffrey RB Jr, Nino-Murcia M, Jorgensen, MJ, Harris DP. Dual-phase helical CT of the liver: value of arterial phase scans in the detection of small (≤1.5 cm) malignant hepatic neoplasms. *AJR* 1995; 164:879–884.

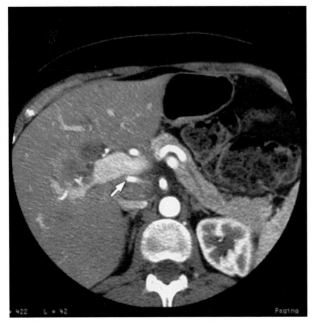

FIG. 117A. CT:arterial phase

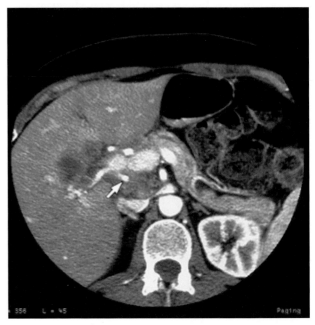

FIG. 117B. CT:arterial phase

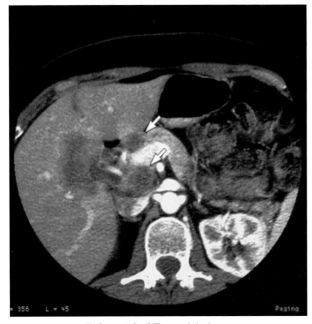

FIG. 117C. CT:arterial phase

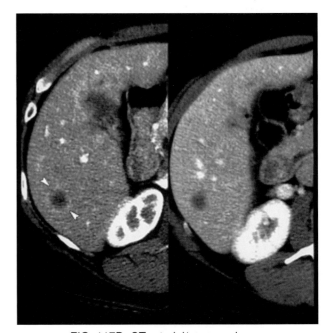

FIG. 117D. CT:arterial/venous phases

History

Outside dynamic CT scan suggests a possible pancreatic mass and liver metastasis. Rule out pancreatic carcinoma.

Findings

Figures 117A–D are arterial-phase images of a biphasic spiral CT scan. Figure 117A demonstrates a normal pancreatic duct. Notice that there is an accessory right hepatic artery seen posterior to the portal vein (arrow). Low-density liver metastases are seen impressing on the portal vein. In addition, there is lymphadenopathy of the portocaval space that is particularly well seen in Figure 117B and C (arrows). A low-density lymph node is also seen, adjacent to the pancreas and anterior to the portal vein (Figure 117 C). Figure 117 D is a side-by-side comparison of arterial- and portal-venous-phase images. During the arterial phase, a low-density liver lesion is noted with an enhancing peripheral rim (arrowheads). The peripheral rim is not evident on the portal-venous-phase images.

Diagnosis

Metastatic adenocarcinoma from an unknown primary tumor. Periportal adenopathy mimicking a pancreatic mass.

Discussion

Thin-section arterial-phase spiral CT clearly identified low-density periportal lymph nodes as the cause of the "mass" seen on the outside study in this case. The pancreatic duct is normal in size and the pancreatic parenchyma enhances normally, thus excluding any intrinsic pancreatic mass. The replaced right hepatic artery was clearly opacified as an enhancing structure in the portocaval space, adjacent to an enlarged lymph node in the portocaval space. The liver metastases were also clearly evident adjacent to the portal vein. The metastasis to the posterior segment of the right lobe seen in Figure 117D clearly demonstrates an enhancing peripheral rim that is not evident on the portal venous phase. This improves the specificity for the diagnosis of metastasis. No known primary tumor was ever found in this patient, who expired 2 months after the CT study.

References

Bluemke DA, Fishman EK. Spiral CT of the liver. *AJR* 1993; 160:787–792.
Zeman RK, Fox SH, Silverman PM, et al. Helical (spiral) CT of the abdomen. *AJR* 1993; 160:719–725.

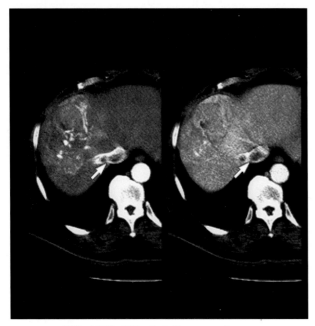

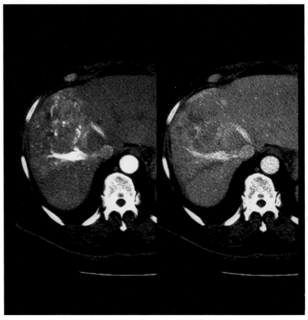

FIG. 118A. CT:arterial/venous phases   FIG. 118B. CT:arterial/venous phases

History

A hypoechoic mass on ultrasound examination. Rule out liver tumor.

Findings

Figures 118A and B are side-by-side comparisons of arterial- and portal-venous–phase scans obtained during a biphasic spiral CT study of the liver. In Figure 118A note the hypervascular mass in the arterial phase that is poorly visualized in the portal-venous phase. Tumor thrombus involving the right hepatic vein and the intrahepatic cava is clearly identified (arrow) on both arterial-and portal-venous–phase images. Note the enlargement of the right hepatic vein and dense opacification in the early arterial phase. Figure 118B again demonstrates diffuse tumor blush within the right lobe of the liver in the arterial phase. The portal venous phase demonstrates only slight heterogeneous attenuation in this area.

Diagnosis

Intrahepatic cholangiocarcinoma with arteriovenous shunting and hepatic venous invasion.

Discussion

The spiral CT features of this lesion mimic hepatocellular carcinoma due to the hypervascularity, arteriovenous shunting, and venous invasion. Although rare, intrahepatic cholangiocarcinomas may be quite large and demonstrate variable degrees of vascularity. Some lesions are necrotic and best visualized in portal-venous–phase images. However, in this patient the lesion was predominantly hypervascular and best identified in the arterial-phase images. Intrahepatic cholangiocarcinomas, when peripheral, may not be associated with dilatation of the biliary tract. Thus, a specific diagnosis is often not possible with imaging studies. The early opacification of the right hepatic vein in the arterial-phase images is diagnostic of arteriovenous shunting. Although commonly noted in hepatocellular carcinoma, it may be demonstrated by other primary or metastatic tumors, as in this case.

References

Hollett MD, Jeffrey RB Jr, Nino-Murcia M, Jorgensen, MJ, harris DP. Dual-phase helical CT of the liver: value of arterial phase scans in the detection of small (≤1.5 cm) malignant hepatic neoplasms. *AJR* 1995; 164:879–884.

Ohashi K, Nakjima Y, Tsutsumi M. Clinical characteristics and proliferating activity of intrahepatic cholangiocarcinoma. *J Gastroenterol Hepatol* 1994; 9:442–446.

Soyer P, Bluemke DA, Hruban RH, Sitzmann JV, Fishmann EK. Intrahepatic cholangiocarcinoma: findings on spiral CT during arterial portography. *Eur J Radiol* 1994; 19:37–42.

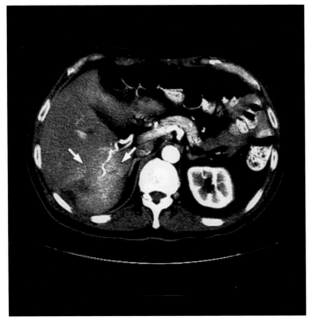

FIG. 121A. CT:arterial phase

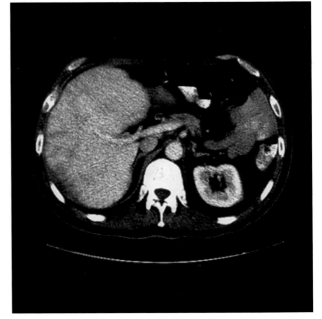

FIG. 121B. CT:venous phase

History

A 56-year-old male, 2 years after resection of a right-lobe metastasis from colon carcinoma.

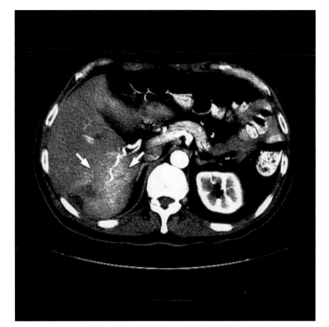

FIG. 121A. CT:arterial phase

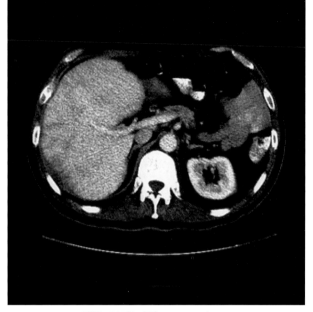

FIG. 121B. CT:venous phase

History

A 56-year-old male, 2 years after resection of a right-lobe metastasis from colon carcinoma.

Findings

Figures 120A and B are arterial-phase scans from a biphasic spiral CT study of the liver. A large, recanalized paraumbilical vein is present, indicating portal hypertension (arrow). The surface of the liver is nodular, which is consistent with cirrhosis. A low-density thrombus is present within the portal vein (arrowhead). Note that there are multiple enhancing tumor nodules. Figure 120C and D are scans obtained during the portal venous phase. In Figure 120C note the extensive portal-venous invasion by tumor. The tumor nodules are not identified on the venous-phase images.

Diagnosis

Multifocal hepatocellular carcinoma identified only on arterial-phase images.

Discussion

Hepatocellular carcinoma derives a robust blood supply from the hepatic artery. Thus, the sensitivity of detection of hepatocellular carcinoma can be substantially improved by dual-phase spiral CT. The sensitivity for detecting primary malignancies in a cirrhotic liver with dynamic CT is only 68%. This is particularly true of satellite nodules, which are often multicentric in distribution. Necrotic lesions, however, will be better seen on portal-venous images. Thus, the combination of the two phases of the examination can not only detect more lesions, but can also characterize the underlying vascularity. The presence of portal-venous invasion generally precludes radical surgery.

References

Hollett MD, Jeffrey RB Jr, Nino-Murcia M, Jorgensen, MJ, Harris DP. Dual-phase helical CT of the liver: value of arterial phase scans in the detection of small (≤1.5 cm) malignant hepatic neoplasms. *AJR* 1995; 164:879–884.

Kihara Y, Tamura S, Kakitsubata S, et al. Optimal timing for delineation of hepatocellular carcinoma in dynamic CT. *J Comput Assist Tomogr* 1993; 17:719–722.

Miller WJ, Baron RL, Dodd GD III, Federle MP. Malignancies in patients with cirrhosis: CT sensitivity and specificity in 200 consecutive transplant patients. *Radiology* 1994; 193:645–650.

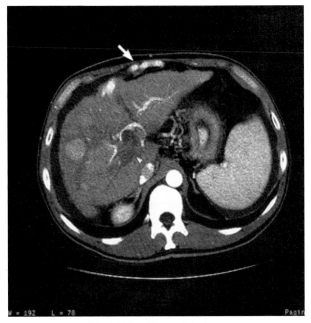

FIG. 120A. CT:arterial phase

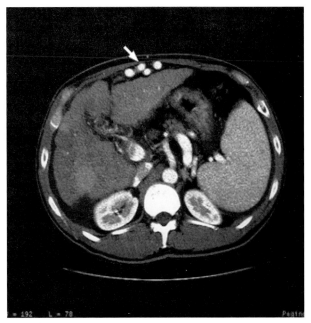

FIG. 120B. CT:arterial phase

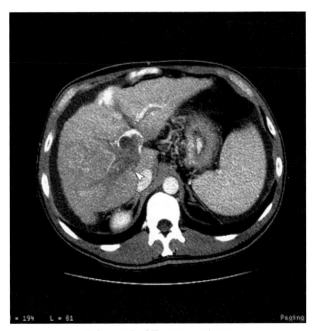

FIG. 120C. CT:venous phase

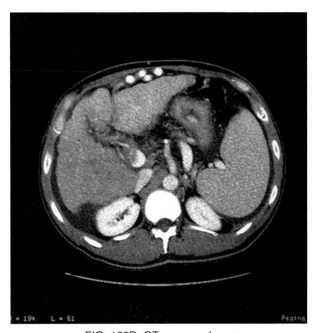

FIG. 120D. CT:venous phase

History

A 51-year-old alcoholic patient with deteriorating liver-function tests.

Findings

Figure 119A is a scan obtained during the early arterial phase of a biphasic spiral CT study of the liver. Notice the wedge-shaped area of increased attenuation in the anterior segment of the right lobe (arrow). This lesion is very difficult to visualize on the portal-venous–phase image (Figure 119B). Figures 119C and D are T1- and T2-weighted images from magnetic resonance imaging (MRI) examination demonstrating no abnormality in the liver.

Diagnosis

Arterial-phase pseudolesion on biphasic spiral CT.

Discussion

Focal areas of increased attenuation may be demonstrated in some normal patients during the early arterial phase of a biphasic spiral CT scan of the liver. The wedge-shaped configuration of this lesion is not characteristic of tumor, which is typically rounded or oval. Similarly, the patient's history of colon cancer also is against the diagnosis of a hypervascular metastasis. Additionally, the normal hepatic MRI scan confirms that there is no evidence of a space-occupying lesion. It is likely that in many instances there are anomalous areas of portal venous drainage in and around the gallbladder fossa, involving the anterior segment of the right lobe and medial segment of the left lobe. These segments may be primarily perfused by the hepatic artery, and thus will appear hyperdense during the arterial phase of a spiral CT scan.

References

Hollett MD, Jeffrey RB Jr, Nino-Murcia M, Jorgensen, MJ, Harris DP. Dual-phase helical CT of the liver: value of arterial phase scans in the detection of small (≤1.5 cm) malignant hepatic neoplasms. *AJR* 1995; 164:879–884.
Yamashita K, Jin M.J, Hirose Y, et al. CT finding of transient focal increased attenuation of the liver adjacent to the gallbladder in acute cholecystitis. *AJR* 1995; 164:343–346.

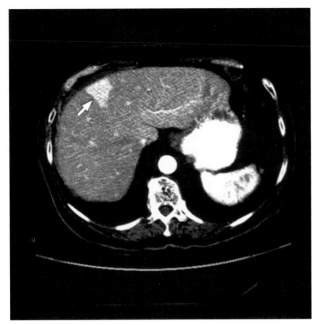

FIG. 119A. CT:arterial phase

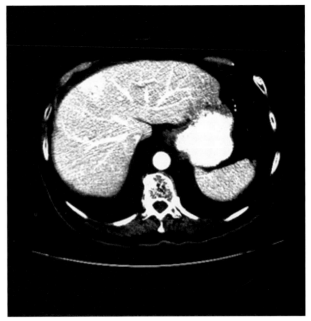

FIG. 119B. CT:venous phase

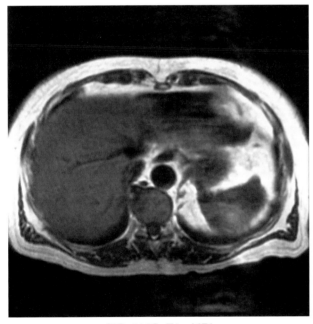

FIG. 119C. T1w MRI

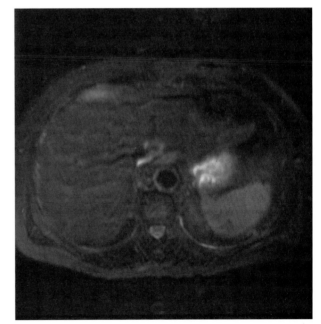

FIG. 119D. T2w MRI

History

Colon carcinoma. Rule out liver metastasis.

Findings

Figures 118A and B are side-by-side comparisons of arterial- and portal-venous–phase scans obtained during a biphasic spiral CT study of the liver. In Figure 118A note the hypervascular mass in the arterial phase that is poorly visualized in the portal-venous phase. Tumor thrombus involving the right hepatic vein and the intrahepatic cava is clearly identified (arrow) on both arterial-and portal-venous–phase images. Note the enlargement of the right hepatic vein and dense opacification in the early arterial phase. Figure 118B again demonstrates diffuse tumor blush within the right lobe of the liver in the arterial phase. The portal venous phase demonstrates only slight heterogeneous attenuation in this area.

Diagnosis

Intrahepatic cholangiocarcinoma with arteriovenous shunting and hepatic venous invasion.

Discussion

The spiral CT features of this lesion mimic hepatocellular carcinoma due to the hypervascularity, arteriovenous shunting, and venous invasion. Although rare, intrahepatic cholangiocarcinomas may be quite large and demonstrate variable degrees of vascularity. Some lesions are necrotic and best visualized in portal-venous–phase images. However, in this patient the lesion was predominantly hypervascular and best identified in the arterial-phase images. Intrahepatic cholangiocarcinomas, when peripheral, may not be associated with dilatation of the biliary tract. Thus, a specific diagnosis is often not possible with imaging studies. The early opacification of the right hepatic vein in the arterial-phase images is diagnostic of arteriovenous shunting. Although commonly noted in hepatocellular carcinoma, it may be demonstrated by other primary or metastatic tumors, as in this case.

References

Hollett MD, Jeffrey RB Jr, Nino-Murcia M, Jorgensen, MJ, harris DP. Dual-phase helical CT of the liver: value of arterial phase scans in the detection of small (≤1.5 cm) malignant hepatic neoplasms. *AJR* 1995; 164:879–884.

Ohashi K, Nakjima Y, Tsutsumi M. Clinical characteristics and proliferating activity of intrahepatic cholangiocarcinoma. *J Gastroenterol Hepatol* 1994; 9:442–446.

Soyer P, Bluemke DA, Hruban RH, Sitzmann JV, Fishmann EK. Intrahepatic cholangiocarcinoma: findings on spiral CT during arterial portography. *Eur J Radiol* 1994; 19:37–42.

Findings

Figure 121A is a scan obtained during the arterial phase of a biphasic spiral CT study of the liver. Note an ill-defined area of increased attenuation (arrows) in the posterior segment of the right lobe in the distribution of the right hepatic artery. Figure 121B is a scan obtained at the same level during the portal venous phase, demonstrating a subtle area of decreased attenuation in the posterior segment of the right lobe. However, no definite lesion is seen in the portal-venous-phase images.

Diagnosis

Arterial phase pseudolesion related to prior hepatic resection.

Discussion

The ill-defined area of increased attenuation identified during the arterial phase in the posterior segment of the right lobe could have been misconstrued as a hypervascular tumor in the absence of an appropriate clinical history. The fact that the patient had colon cancer militates against the diagnosis of a hypervascular tumor. In addition, the area of abnormality is within the segment of the prior surgery. A scan performed 1 year later revealed no evidence of tumor. It is likely that the surgical procedure, in some fashion, altered the hepatic blood flow to the posterior segment of the right lobe. Therefore, with hypovascular tumors, one must be cautious in interpreting flow defects in areas of prior surgical resection. In some instances, flow defects in arterial-phase perfusion may mimic tumors, as in this case.

References

Bluemke DA, Fishman EK. Spiral CT of the liver. *AJR* 1993;160:787–792.

Herts BR, Einstein DM, Paushter DM. Spiral CT of the abdomen: artifacts and potential pitfalls. *AJR* 1993; 161:1185–1190.

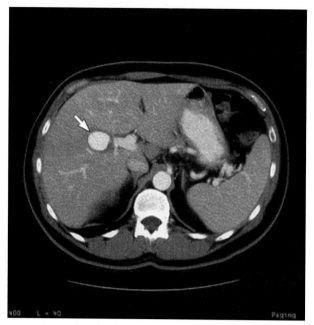

FIG. 122A. Contrast-enhanced CT

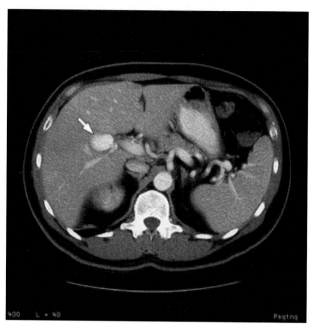

FIG. 122B. Contrast-enhanced CT

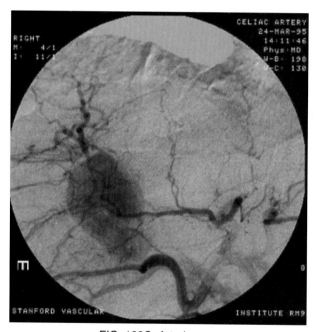

FIG. 122C. Arteriogram

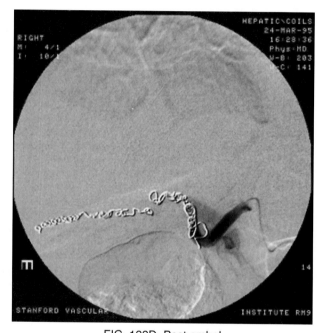

FIG. 122D. Post embol

History

Fever of unknown origin and increased liver function test valves.

Findings

Figures 122A and B are contrast-enhanced spiral CT scans of the liver. A mycotic aneurysm with intense enhancement is seen immediately adjacent to the undivided portion of the right portal vein (arrow). The anterior segment of the right portal vein is occluded by the mycotic aneurysm. Figures 122C and D are from a hepatic arterial embolization. Note the large mycotic aneurysm in Figure 122C. Following embolization (Figure 122D) there is no filling of the mycotic aneurysm.

Diagnosis

Mycotic aneurysm of the hepatic artery secondary to bacterial endocarditis.

Discussion

This patient ultimately proved to have subacute bacterial endocarditis with blood cultures positive for *staphylococcus aureus*. Echocardiography demonstrated multiple vegetations on the mitral valve. The patient was asymptomatic except for persistent fever. The spiral CT clearly identified the mycotic aneurysm and its proximity to the portal vein. These lesions are often very treacherous to approach surgically, and are best treated by angiographic embolization. This was successfully performed, and the patient made an uneventful recovery.

Mycotic aneurysms of the liver are very rare except in patients with bacterial endocarditis. They may involve the upper abdominal aorta from T12 to L3. These aneurysms may cause back pain when there is hemorrhage into the paraortic tissues. Most pseudoaneurysms of the hepatic artery result from pancreatitis, trauma, vasculitis, or interventional biliary procedures.

References

Khoda J, Lantsberg L, Sebbag G. Hepatic artery mycotic aneurysm as a cause of hemobilia. *J Hepatol* 1993; 17:131–132.

Rogers DW, Lumeng L, Goulet RJ, Canal DR. Ruptured mycotic pseudoaneurysm of the gastroduodenal artery presenting with hemoperitoneum and subcapsular liver hematoma. *Digest Dis Sci* 1990; 35:661–664.

Sanchez-Bueno F, Robles R, Ramirez P. Hepatic artery complications after liver transplantation. *Clin Transplant* 1994; 8:399–404.

The Musculoskeletal System

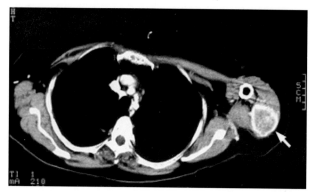

FIG. 123A. Contrast-enhanced CT

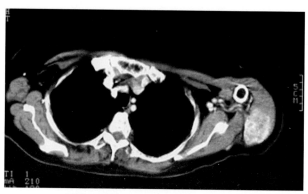

FIG. 123B. Contrast-enhanced CT

History

A 73-year-old female with a history of a left nephrectomy for renal-cell carcinoma. A CT scan was obtained for evaluation of the patient's increasing left shoulder pain, as well as to determine the extent of possible metastatic disease in the chest.

Findings

A spiral CT scan with soft-tissue windows demonstrates an enhancing mass in the left deltoid muscle. There is a peripheral rim of enhancement clearly defined (arrow). On lung windows (not shown), multiple lung metastases were also seen.

Diagnosis

Metastatic carcinoma to muscle from the patient's primary renal-cell carcinoma.

Discussion

Metastases from primary tumors to the musculoskeletal system are typically represented by lytic, blastic, or mixed-type bony lesions. However, metastases to the subcutaneous tissues or muscle are rare and are often overlooked on radiologic studies. With the advent of spiral CT with properly timed injections to ensure study optimization, masses within muscle should be easier to define, particularly if the lesions are vascular.

The most common primary tumors that result in muscle metastases are those of the lung, colon, and pancreas. Other tumors, including breast, kidney, and lymphoma, can also cause muscle involvement. The size and appearance of metastatic tumor to muscle is variable, ranging in size from 1 cm to over 10 cm. These lesions, as documented on spiral CT, are often hypervascular as compared to normal muscle, which enhances only minimally. Also, an enhancing rim or enhancing pseudocapsule is often seen in these cases.

In this case, the patient's primary tumor was a renal-cell carcinoma, and it is not uncommon for both the primary tumor and renal-cell metastases in this disease to be very vascular. The differential diagnosis of this lesion would include a metastatic tumor and a primary tumor of muscle, including lymphoma, leiomyosarcoma, and malignant fibrous histiocytoma. Although a primary tumor is considered, it would be less likely on the basis of the clinical history alone.

Enhancing musculoskeletal lesions with peripheral rim enhancement are not uncommonly seen in inflammatory disease. However, in those cases the entire lesion will typically not enhance. We have found that with intramuscular abscesses showing rim enhancement, there is typically more of an inflammatory process around the lesion, whereas with metastatic foci there is often very sharp margination. Obviously, the clinical history and presentation can be helpful in distinguishing the two possibilities. In most cases of metastases to muscle, the patient has a known primary tumor and the muscle lesion may represent either an area of relapse or metastatic disease. However, in other cases the muscle metastases may actually be the initial site of disease presentation. We have seen at least one case in which the patient's presentation was back and rib pain, and in which a metastasis to the left paraspinal muscle was noted in what was subsequently proven to be a lung cancer.

References

Resnick D, Niwayama G, Skeletal metastases. In: Resnick D. (ed.): *Diagnosis of Bone and Joint Disorders.* Philadelphia: WB Saunders, 1995, Ch 85, pp. 4039–4043.

Sridhar KS, Rao RK, Kunhardt B. Skeletal muscle metastases from lung cancer. *Cancer* 1987; 59:1530–1534.

Torosian MH, Botet JF, Paglia M. Colon carcinoma metastatic to the thigh an unusual site of metastasis. Report of a case. *Dis Colon Rectum* 1987; 30:805–808.

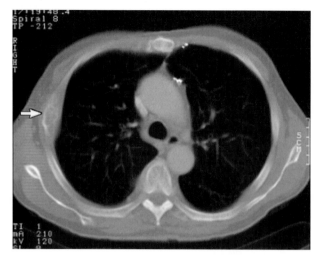

FIG. 124A. Contrast-enhanced CT

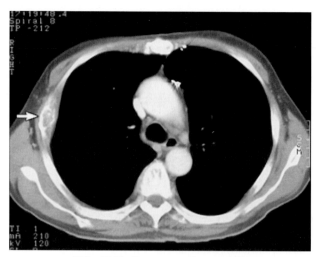

FIG. 124B. Contrast-enhanced CT

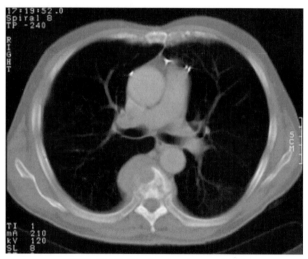

FIG. 124C. Contrast-enhanced CT

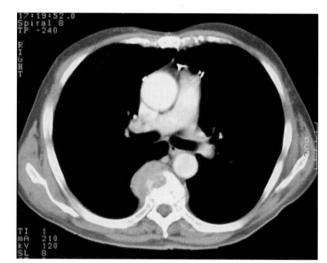

FIG. 124D. Contrast-enhanced CT

History

A 71-year-old male with symptoms caused by weight loss and low-grade fever. A chest x-ray suggested possible lung or pleural based masses. A spiral CT scan was done for evaluation.

Findings

The CT scan demonstrates evidence of lytic lesions in several right ribs and in the thoracic spine. The lesions in both locations are associated with a soft-tissue mass, and particularly the spinal lesion at approximately the T5–T6 level. Destruction of bone was seen in a predominantly lytic pattern.

Diagnosis

Hodgkin disease of the spine and ribs.

Discussion

Primary lymphoma of bone is rare and accounts for approximately 5% of all primary bone tumors. Secondary involvement, however, is common in both Hodgkin and non-Hodgkin lymphoma. In a series by Rosenberg et al., osseous involvement was found in 16% of cases during the course of disease. The prevalence of bone involvement is higher in children, with up to 25% having bone lesions. Bone involvement is more common in Hodgkin than non-Hodgkin lymphoma, with the most frequent areas of involvement being the spine, pelvis, and skull.

In Hodgkin disease, tumors may arise (either through hematogenous dissemination or contiguous spread) from adjacent lymph nodes. Tumor patterns may be osteosclerotic, osteolytic, or of a mixed pattern. Sclerotic lesions, however, account for 45% of all bone lesions in Hodgkin disease.

At present, spiral CT is the gold standard for staging lymphoma. Therefore, one should look carefully at the musculoskeletal system to detect any involvement. If there is bone involvement in addition to other sites of disease, the patient has is stage IV disease. In addition to skeletal involvement, lymphoma may involve muscle, subcutaneous tissues, or skin. In select cases, lymphoma is primary in an extremity and may be difficult to distinguish from other primary bone tumors, including fibrosarcoma or metastatic disease.

References

Buerger LF, Monteleone DN. Leukemic-lymphomatous infiltration of skeletal muscle: systematic study of 82 autopsy cases. *Cancer* 1966; 19:1416–1422.

Fishman EK, Kuhlman JE, Jones RJ. CT of lymphoma: spectrum of disease. *RadioGraphics* 1991; 11:647–669.

Malloy PC, Fishman EK, Magid D. Lymphoma of bone, muscle, and skin: CT findings. *AJR* 1992; 159:805–809.

Rosenberg SA, Diamond HD, Taslowitz B, Craver CF. Lymphosarcoma: review of 1269 cases. *Medicine* 1961; 40:31–84.

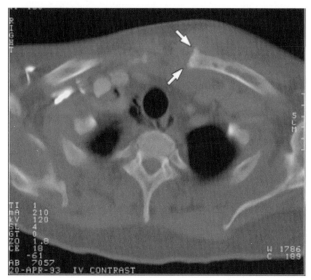

FIG. 125A. Contrast-enhanced CT

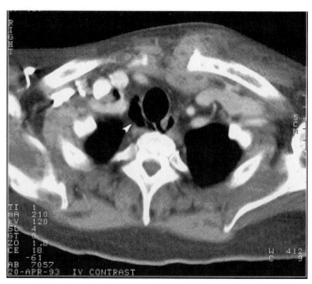

FIG. 125B. Contrast-enhanced CT

History

A 62-year-old male with a history of rheumatoid arthritis treated with prednisone. The patient had a history of swallowing difficulties and esophagitis secondary to *Candida* infection. The dose of prednisone was raised to 60 mg 2 days before admission. The patient presented with fever and sternoclavicular-joint swelling and pain.

Findings

A spiral CT scan using 4-mm thick sections reconstructed at 2-mm intervals demonstrates marked inflammation of the left sternoclavicular joint. There is also evidence of erosion of the clavicular head (arrows). Associated inflammation of the left pectoralis major muscle is also noted, and air is seen in the mediastinum (arrowhead).

Diagnosis

Osteomyelitis of the left sternoclavicular joint.

Discussion

Spiral CT combining rapid contrast-medium infusion and narrow collimation is ideal for the evaluation of musculoskeletal infection. Spiral CT helps define the compartment of involvement as well as the extent of involvement. Although magnetic resonance imaging (MRI) is the dominant study for musculoskeletal pathology, spiral CT has certain specific applications, in which it has proven very successful.

With standard CT imaging, evaluation of sternoclavicular joints may be difficult because of interscan or intrascan motion. Spiral CT routinely allows high-quality images to be obtained without patient motion, which is important if multiplanar or three-dimensional images are to be obtained. We previously reported a series of seven patients with suspected infection of the sternoclavicular joints who had spiral CT scanning. All cases were successfully completed without any interscan or intrascan motion. In six cases infection of the sternoclavicular joint was found, which in five cases included osteomyelitis of the clavicular head. The CT scans were used for patient-management decisions, and in select cases subsequent scans were obtained for follow-up.

In cases of musculoskeletal infection, the use of contrast enhancement helps to optimize detection of the inflammatory process. All muscles enhance, but typically inflamed or infected areas will enhance to a lesser degree, making involvement more detectable. Magnetic resonance imaging (MRI), however, is often better at defining the full extent of muscle involvement, although in most cases CT will suffice.

References

Fishman EK, Wyatt SH, Bluemke DA, Urban BA. Spiral CT of musculoskeletal pathology: preliminary observations. *Skeletal Radiol* 1993; 22:253–256.

Linthoudt D, Velan F, Ott H. Abscess formation in sternoclavicular joint septic arthritis. *Rheumatology* 1989; 16:413–414.

Tecce, PM, Fishman EK. Spiral CT with multiplanar reconstruction in the diagnosis of sternoclavicular osteomyelitis. *Skeletal Radiol* 1995; 24:275–281.

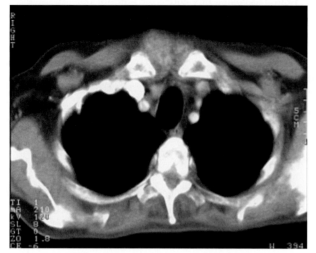

FIG. 126A. Contrast-enhanced CT

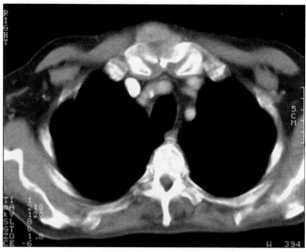

FIG. 126B. Contrast-enhanced CT

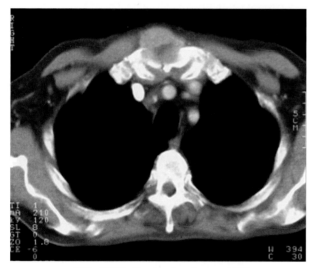

FIG. 126C. Contrast-enhanced CT

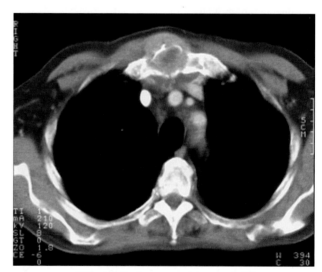

FIG. 126D. Contrast-enhanced CT

History

A 72-year-old male with a history of both bladder cancer and lymphoma. The patient presented with sternal pain and a palpable mass.

Findings

A spiral CT scan of the chest demonstrates a 2 × 3 × 5-cm mass extending above the anterior portion of the sternum. No evidence of adenopathy is seen and no evidence of lung metastases is noted in this examination.

Diagnosis

Metastatic, poorly differentiated carcinoma consistent with the patient's primary bladder cancer.

Discussion

Although bone scans remain the primary modality for the detection of skeletal metastases, metastatic disease to bone is well defined by spiral CT scanning. In cases of lung cancer, special attention is paid to the ribs and spine to rule out direct tumor extension or metastatic disease. In the present case, there is a large sternal mass with bone destruction. Since the patient does have a history of primary tumor, metastases would obviously be at the top of the differential diagnosis list. However, a primary tumor such as a plasmacytoma cannot be excluded on the basis of CT findings alone. Once the tumor was biopsied, however, the diagnosis of metastases from the patient's bladder carcinoma became clear.

Evaluation of the sternum had been shown to be optimized with CT scanning, often supplemented by two- and three-dimensional reconstruction. Because the sternum lies in an oblique plane, it is very easy to overlook tumor or inflammatory disease on routine radiographs. CT scanning provides an optimal view of the sternum, and processes that cause destruction are therefore easily documented. This is true whether one is looking at inflammatory disease or neoplastic disease.

When evaluating bone, it is important that careful attention be paid to technique. Images made with a bone algorithm tend to be helpful, particularly in looking at early changes in the cortex or medullary region. It is especially helpful to obtain thin sections with narrow collimation when reconstruction of data sets is needed. Finally, the use of intravenous infusion of contrast medium should be considered in cases in which suspected metastatic or primary tumor is to be evaluated. In this case, the use of contrast enhancement better defines the full extent of disease and accentuates tumor infiltrating bone.

References

Fishman EK. "Spiral CT evaluation of the musculoskeletal system." In: Fishman EK, Jeffrey RB Jr (eds.): *Spiral CT: Principles, Techniques and Clinical Application.* New York: Raven Press, 1995, pp. 141–158.

Magid D. Two-dimensional and three dimensional computed tomographic imaging in musculoskeletal tumors. *Radiol Clin North Am* 1993; 31:425–447.

Pretorius ES, Fishman EK. Helical (spiral) CT of the musculoskeletal system. *Radiol Clin North Am* 1995; 33:949–979.

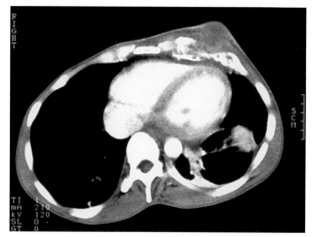

FIG. 127A. Contrast-enhanced CT

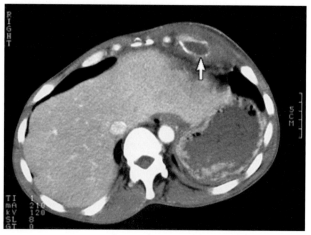

FIG. 127B. Contrast-enhanced CT

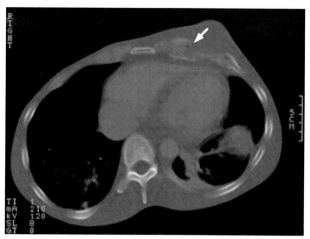

FIG. 127C. Contrast-enhanced CT

History

A 40-year-old male with a history of acquired immune deficiency syndrome (AIDS) and active intravenous drug abuse. The patient presented with a rapidly enlarging, painful left-chest-wall mass. The patient noted that he began having pain in this region several months earlier. The clinical diagnosis included neoplastic and inflammatory processes.

Findings

A spiral CT scan demonstrates a large soft-tissue mass involving the left anterior chest wall, with underlying rib destruction (arrow). The clinical history suggests an inflammatory process.

Diagnosis

Pseudomonas osteomyelitis involving the 6th and 7th ribs, with associated abscess formation.

Discussion

The patient with human immunodeficiency virus (HIV) infection has a decrease in host-defense mechanisms predisposing to a wide range of inflammatory and neoplastic diseases. Several articles have recently discussed the musculoskeletal complications of AIDS, including osteomyelitis, myositis, and lymphoma. Steinbach et al. reviewed a series of 45 HIV-positive patients with musculoskeletal disease. Of these, 15 patients had osteomyelitis. The causes of the osteomyelitis varied from *Nocardia* to *Cryptococcus neoformans* and bacillary angiomatosis. We also previously reported our experience with the spectrum of disease in the AIDS patient. In many cases, inflammatory and neoplastic processes can have a similar appearance.

Spiral CT is often used in the HIV-positive patient for evaluation of processes suspected from physical examination or clinical presentation. In the present case, the clinical differential diagnosis was between a neoplastic and an inflammatory process. Spiral CT with contrast enhancement demonstrated the destructive lesion in bone, with an associated soft-tissue mass consistent with infection. A neoplasm was considered, but because of the area of low density within the mass, and its general appearance, infection was felt to be the most likely cause.

The detection of intramuscular processes and evaluation of their extent are best done with intravenous contrast enhancement. Many abscesses will have peripheral enhancement. There is a definite differential enhancement between normal muscle and infectious tissue. In cases with intramuscular abscess, we have also found it helpful to perform several delayed scans through the area in question. In certain cases, the peripheral enhancement is best seen on delayed scans, and areas of central necrosis become more seen on delayed scans, and areas of central necrosis is become more obvious at approximately 10 to 20 minutes after the initial injection.

In HIV-positive patients, musculoskeletal tumors that occur with an increased frequency include lymphoma, particularly non-Hodgkin lymphoma, and Kaposi sarcoma. CT and magnetic resonance imaging (MRI) appear to be the studies of choice for evaluating these patients, with the choice of specific imaging modality depending on multiple factors, including the time necessary to perform the examination, because imaging is often done in an acutely ill patient who is not very cooperative. In this case, a 32 to 40 second spiral CT scan may be the ideal study.

References

1. Steinbach LS, Tehranzadeh J, Fleckenstein JL, Vanarthos WJ, Pais MJ. Human immunodeficiency virus infection: musculoskeletal manifestations. *Radiology* 1993; 186:833–838.
2. Magid D, Fishman EK. Musculoskeletal infections in patients with AIDS: CT findings. *AJR* 1992; 158:603–607.
3. Safai B, Diaz B, Schwartz J. Malignant neoplasms associated with human immunodeficiency virus infection. *Cancer* 1992; 42:74–95.

The Pancreas

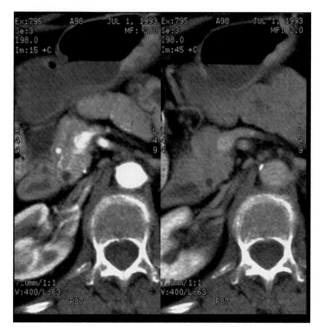

FIG. 128A. CT:arterial/venous phases

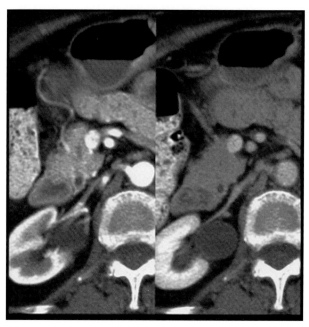

FIG. 128B. CT:arterial/venous phases

History

Vague midepigastric pain and weight loss. Rule out pancreatic carcinoma.

Findings

Figures 128A and B are side-by-side comparisons of the normal pancreas during both arterial- and portal-venous-phase imaging. Notice during the arterial phase that there is intense enhancement of the pancreatic parenchyma, with ex-cellent delineation of the peripancreatic vasculature. In the portal venous phase there is washout of contrast material from the pancreas and relatively poor opacification of arterial structures.

Diagnosis

Normal biphasic spiral CT scan of the pancreas.

Discussion

As in biphasic spiral CT scanning of the liver, arterial-phase imaging of the pancreas affords a number of diagnostic advantages. When combined with the rapid-bolus technique (5 ml/sec for a total of 150 ml of 60% contrast medium) there is often significantly improved pancreatic enhancement during early-phase images (obtained approximately 25 to 30 seconds after initiation of the bolus). Studies have shown that the mean enhancement of the normal pancreas is 82 HU during the arterial phase and 62 HU (25% less) during the portal venous phase. Arterial-phase images have the advantage of demonstrating hypervascular lesions (neuroendocrine tumors) and identifying small hypovascular tumors (ductal adenocarcinoma) as compared to the normally enhancing pancreas. In addition, small peripancreatic arteries are routinely better visualized during arterial-phase imaging. This enables more confident diagnosis of arterial encasement. However, portal-venous-phase images are essential to diagnose venous obstruction and hepatic metastasis, since these are often less well seen during the arterial phase.

The initial arterial phase in spiral CT of the pancreas is generally performed with collimation of 3 to 5 mm. This can be accomplished with a pitch of 1 to 1.5. Overlapping reconstructions are used to avoid misregistration artifacts. Anomalous arteries can be identified, which may be of particular value to the operating surgeon if major pancreatic resection is considered.

References

Dupuy DE, Costello P, Ecker CP. Spiral CT of the pancreas. *Radiology* 1992; 183:815–818.

Fishman EK, Wyatt SH, Ney DR, et al. Spiral CT of the pancreas with multiplanar display. *AJR* 1992; 159:1209–1215.

Hollett MD, Jorgensen MJ, Jeffrey RB Jr. Quantitative evaluation of pancreatic enhancement during dual-phase helical CT. *Radiology* 1995; 195:363–370.

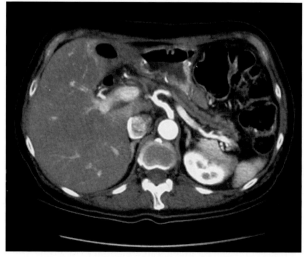

FIG. 129A. CT:arterial phase

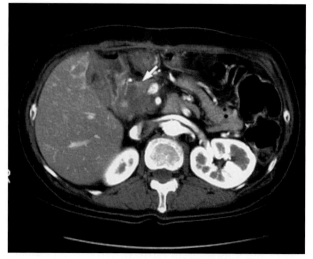

FIG. 129B. CT:arterial phase

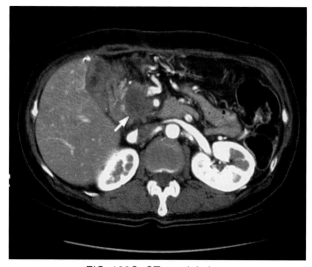

FIG. 129C. CT:arterial phase

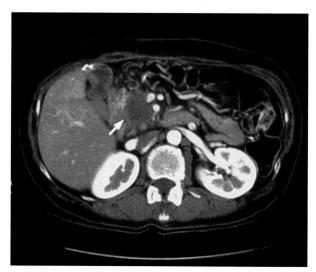

FIG. 129D. CT:arterial phase

History

Midepigastric pain and weight loss. Rule out pancreatic carcinoma.

Findings

Figures 129A–D are scans obtained during the arterial phase of a biphasic spiral CT study of the pancreas. Note in Figure 129A that there is excellent opacification of the celiac and splenic arteries. The distal pancreas is quite atrophic, and there is dilatation of the pancreatic duct. Figures 129B and C demonstrate a low-density mass (arrow) in the head and neck of the pancreas, with encasement of a replaced right hepatic artery originating from the superior mesenteric artery. Figure 129D demonstrates a large mass in the pancreatic head (arrow) with encasement of a posterior branch coming off the superior mesenteric artery, probably representing the posterior inferior pancreatic duodenal artery.

Diagnosis

Pancreatic carcinoma with arterial encasement.

Discussion

Use of the rapid-bolus technique (5 ml/sec) provides excellent vascular opacification during the arterial phase. Thin collimation (3 mm) optimizes the spatial resolution of the pancreas and surrounding fat planes. One of the most common variants of splanchnic arterial anatomy is a replaced right hepatic artery coming from the superior mesenteric artery. This variant is clearly evident in this patient, as is also the tumor encasement around this vessel. The inferior pancreatic duodenal arcades are rarely visualized with standard portal-venous CT scans. In this patient, however, this small vessel was demonstrated along with the adjacent tumor encasement.

References

Dupuy DE, Costello P, Ecker CP. Spiral CT of the pancreas. *Radiology* 1992; 183:815–818.

Fishman EK, Wyatt SH, Ney DR, et al. Spiral CT of the pancreas with multiplanar display. *AJR* 1992; 159:1209–1215.

Hollett MD, Jorgensen MJ, Jeffrey RB Jr. Quantitative evaluation of pancreatic enhancement during dual-phase helical CT. *Radiology* 1995; 195:363–370.

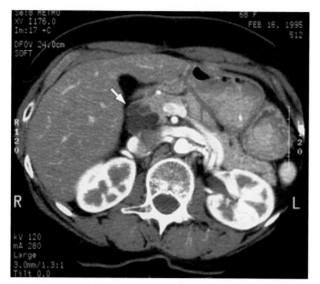

FIG. 130A. CT:arterial phase]

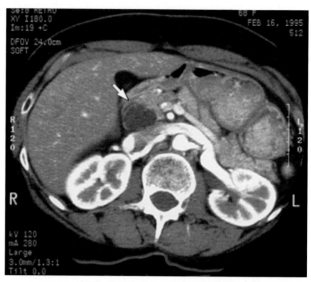

FIG. 130B. CT:arterial phase

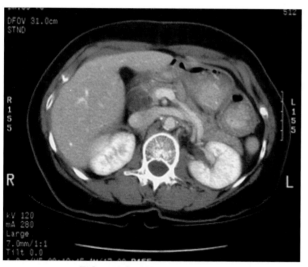

FIG. 130C. CT:venous phase

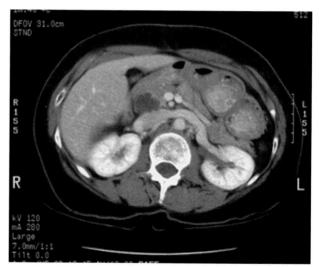

FIG. 130D. CT:venous phase

History

Pancreatic cyst on sonography. Rule out cystic neoplasm in this 47-year-old female.

Findings

Figures 130A and B are arterial-phase images taken from a biphasic spiral CT study of the pancreas. Notice the septated cystic mass in the head of the pancreas (arrow). Figures 130C and D are scans obtained during the portal venous phase providing similar information. Note the lack of mural tissue within the mass. A few small, thin septations are noted within the mass.

Diagnosis

Cystadenoma of the pancreas.

Discussion

In adult patients without a history of pancreatitis, cystic masses in the pancreas should be considered neoplasms until proven otherwise. The hallmark of mucinous cystadenocarcinoma is a complex cystic mass containing solid mural tissue and thick septations. In this patient only thin septations were noted, without mural nodularity. At surgery, a benign pancreatic mucinous cystadenoma was resected. Recent studies suggest that it might be possible to differentiate various pancreatic cystic masses with fine-needle aspiration cytology and fluid aspiration.

References

Ros PR, Hamrick-Turner JE, Chiechi MV, Ros LH, Gallego P, Burton SS. Cystic masses of the pancreas. *RadioGraphics* 1992; 12:673.

Soyer P, Rabenandrasana A, Van Beers B, et al. Cystic tumors of the pancreas: dynamic CT studies. *J Comput Assist Tomogr* 1004; 18:420.

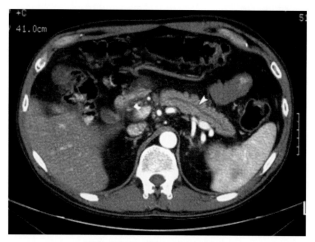

FIG. 131A. CT:arterial phase

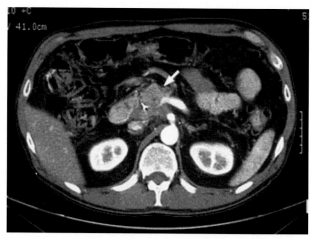

FIG. 131B. CT:arterial phase

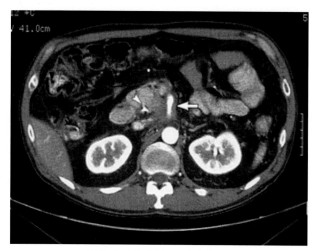

FIG. 131C. CT:arterial phase

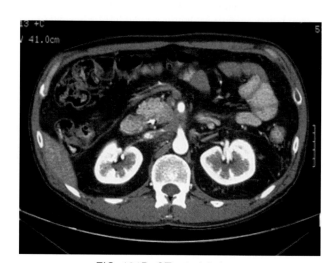

FIG. 131D. CT:arterial phase

History

Weight loss and back pain. Rule out pancreatic carcinoma.

Findings

Figures 131A–D are scans obtained during the arterial phase of a biphasic spiral CT scan. Notice the excellent visualization of the peripancreatic vasculature and the intense enhancement of the pancreatic parenchyma. The pancreatic duct is identified in Figure 131A (arrowhead), and is mildly dilated. In Figure 131B a large mass is identified in the body of the pancreas, encasing the splenic vein (arrow). Superior mesenteric artery encasement is clearly depicted in Figures 131C and D (arrow). There is a high-attenuation endoprosthesis in the common bile duct (arrowhead, Figure 131C).

Diagnosis

Pancreatic carcinoma with arterial and venous encasement.

Discussion

Arterial-phase images in biphasic spiral CT of the pancreas are often quite helpful in diagnosing arterial encasement. In this patient the extension of tumor along the superior mesenteric artery was critical in the decision not to perform radical pancreatic surgery. Stenosis of the portal vein by the tumor was also clearly evident, even on the arterial-phase images. In many patients with pancreatic carcinoma, high-resolution scans can be obtained with 3-mm collimation. Often these patients have experienced significant weight loss, and image quality is enhanced by thin-slice collimation. Posterior extension of pancreatic carcinoma to involve the splanchnic vessel is typical of this disease, and is associated with a very poor prognosis.

References

Fishman EK, Wyatt SH, Ney DR, Kuhlman JE, Siegelman SS. Spiral CT of the pancreas with multiplanar display. *AJR* 1992; 159:1209–1215.

Hollett MD, Jorgensen MJ, Jeffrey RB Jr. Quantitative evaluation of pancreatic enhancement during dual-phase helical CT. *Radiology* 1995; 195:363–370.

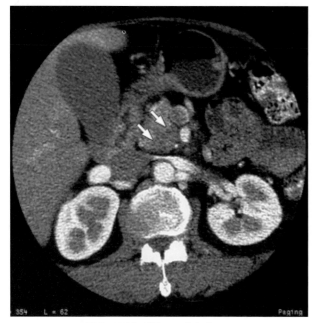

FIG. 132A. CT:arterial phase

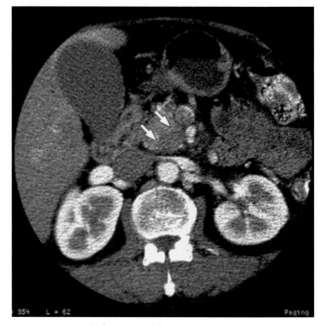

FIG. 132B. CT:arterial phase

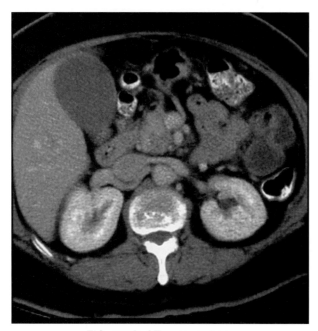

FIG. 132C. CT:venous phase

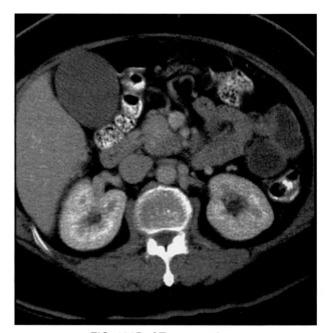

FIG. 132D. CT:venous phase

History

Pancreatic mass identified on an outside sonogram. Rule out carcinoma.

Findings

Figures 132A and B are arterial-phase images from a biphasic spiral CT study of the pancreas. Note the low-attenuation mass in the uncinate process of the pancreas (arrow). In addition, there is a low-density "filling defect" in the superior mesenteric vein. Figure 132C and D are scans obtained during the portal venous phase demonstrating patency of the superior mesenteric vein without evidence of intraluminal thrombus.

Diagnosis

Pancreatic carcinoma. Flow defect in the superior mesenteric vein simulating thrombosis.

Discussion

Arterial-phase images of the upper abdomen may result in a variety of flow-related artifacts in the major veins. This is due to mixing of opacified and unopacified blood. The most common site of these artifacts is the inferior cava at the level of the renal veins. Unopacified blood returning from the lower extremities is mixed with blood from the kidneys, resulting in a mottled appearance that may simulate intraluminal thrombus. In this patient with a pancreatic carcinoma, the flow defect was confirmed on the follow-up portal vein images as not being due to thrombus. It is important to carefully evaluate venous structures on images acquired during the portal venous phase, in order to avoid potential misdiagnosis of flow-related artifacts.

References

Freeny PC, Traverso LW, Ryan JA. Diagnosis and staging of pancreatic adenocarcinoma with dynamic computed tomography. *Am J Surg* 1993; 165:600–606.

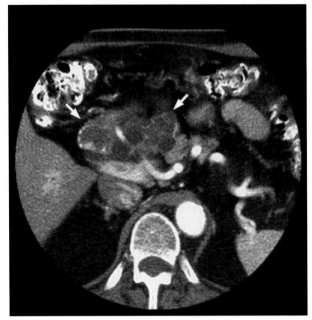

FIG. 133A. CT:arterial phase

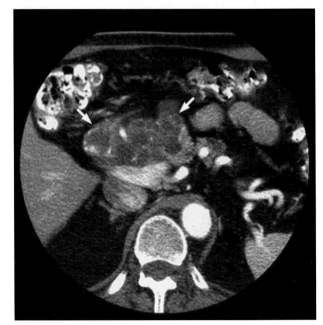

FIG. 133B. CT:arterial phase

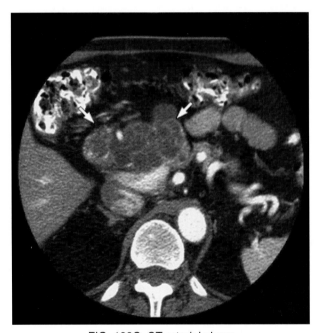

FIG. 133C. CT:arterial phase

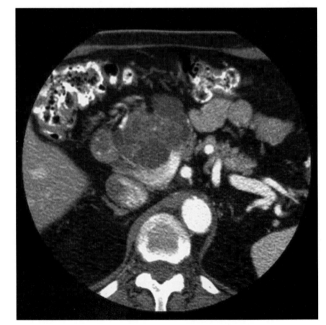

FIG. 133D. CT:arterial phase

History

Pancreatic cystic mass noted on an outside sonogram. Rule out cystic neoplasm in this 75-year-old male.

282

Findings

Figures 133A–D are scans obtained during the arterial phase of a biphasic spiral CT study of the pancreas. Note the thin enhancing septa within the cystic mass seen in the neck of the pancreas (arrows). In Figures 133A and B the hepatic artery is identified adjacent to the mass, without evidence of encasement. The low-density cystic locules of the mass appear to be quite small; in many of the images they are less than a centimeter in size.

Diagnosis

Microcystic adenoma of the pancreas.

Discussion

The arterial-phase images in this case demonstrated small cystic locules within the mass and enhancing septa between the locules. These features are characteristic of microcystic adenoma, which is a benign lesion containing serous fluid. These lesions may calcify and their central septa may have a rather striking degree of enhancement. Unlike mucinous cystadenocarcinomas, the cystic locules within these lesions are often microscopic. When visible they are typically less than 2 cm in size. Mucinous ceptic neoplasmas are characterized by mural nodularity or tumor neovascularity within thickened septa within the mass. The locules typically are greater than 2 cm in size. Both lesions may contain calcifications.

References

Ros PR, Hamrick-Turner JE, Chiechi MV, Ros LH, Gallego P, Burton SS. Cystic masses of the pancreas. *RadioGraphics* 1992; 12:673.

Soyer P, Rabenandrasana A, Van Beers B, et al. Cystic tumors of the pancreas: dynamic CT studies. *J Comput Assist Tomogr* 1004; 18:420.

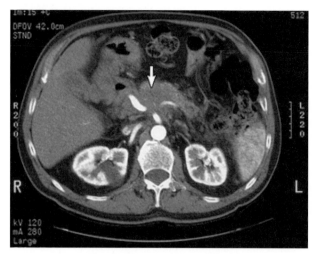

FIG. 134A. CT:arterial phase]

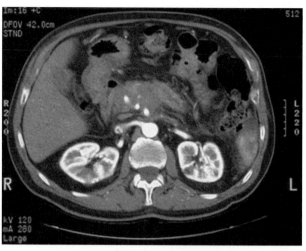

FIG. 134B. CT:arterial phase

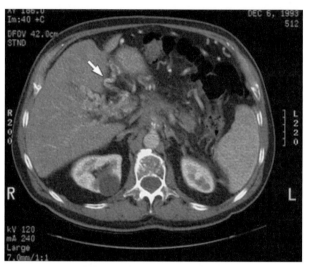

FIG. 134C. CT:venous phase

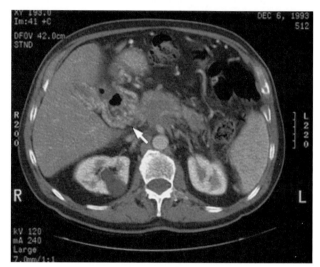

FIG. 134D. CT:venous phase

History

A 73-year-old male with a suspected pancreatic lesion on ultrasound examination.

Findings

Figures 134A and B are arterial-phase scans of a biphasic spiral CT scan of the pancreas. Note the extensive encasement of the celiac axis by the pancreatic tumor (arrow). In Figure 134B there is encasement of the superior mesenteric artery as well. Figures 134C and D are scans obtained during the portal venous phase of the study demonstrating lack of visualization of the splenic vein and extensive periportal varices (arrow) due to portal vein occlusion. Prominent gallbladder varices are noted.

Diagnosis

Pancreatic carcinoma with arterial encasement and venous occlusion.

Discussion

In this patient the arterial-phase images clearly demonstrated extensive encasement of the celial and superior mesenteric arteries. However, splenic-vein obstruction was best assessed during the later portal venous phase of the scan. In this patient enlarged gastroepiploic veins were demonstrated, as a result of splenic-vein occlusion. In addition, numerous periportal collaterals were evident as a result of obstruction of the portal vein. Because of extensive tumor involvement, the patient was not considered for surgery and was treated with radiation and chemotherapy. The patient died, however, within 2 months after therapy was begun.

References

Dupuy DE, Costello P, Ecker CP. Spiral CT of the pancreas. *Radiology* 1992; 183:815–818.

Fishman EK, Wyatt SH, Ney DR, et al. Spiral CT of the pancreas with multiplanar display. *AJR* 1992; 159:1209–1215.

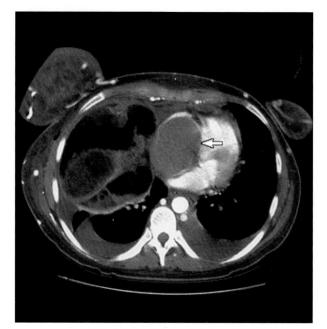

FIG. 135A. CT:arterial phase]

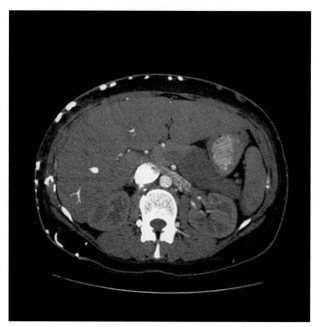

FIG. 135B. CT:arterial phase

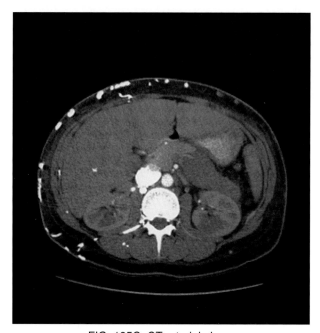

FIG. 135C. CT:arterial phase

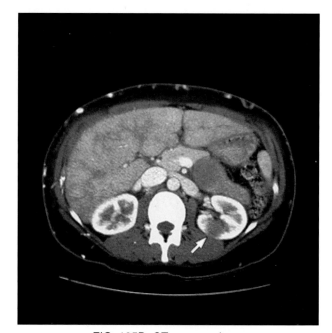

FIG. 135D. CT:venous phase

History

A 33-year-old female with shortness of breath and a mass on chest x-ray. Rule out abdominal abnormality.

Findings

Figure 135A is a scan of the thorax obtained during the arterial phase of a biphasic spiral CT examination. An incidental fatty mass within the right thorax is noted, which was a benign mediastinal teratoma. However, there is a soft-tissue mass filling almost the entire right atrium (arrow). Figure 135B is a scan during the arterial phase of the upper abdomen, demonstrating extensive subcutaneous venous collaterals and dense opacification of the inferior vena cava due to collateral intracostal lumbar veins. Figure 135C is an arterial-phase image demonstrating decreased attenuation of the distal portion of the pancreas. A vague low-density mass is evident in the left kidney. Figure 135D is a scan obtained during the portal venous phase after a 65-second delay, demonstrating a more discrete rounded mass in the tail of the pancreas. Note also a low-density mass in the left kidney (arrow).

Diagnosis

Pancreatic and renal non-Hodgkin lymphoma.

Discussion

Biphasic spiral CT of the abdomen requires a relatively normal cardiac output and circulation time. The obstructing mass in the right atrium in the present case resulted in poor opacification of the liver and pancreas during the arterial phase, which was obtained at approximately 25 to 55 seconds after the initiation of the bolus injection of contrast medium. Delayed images more precisely depicted the true extent of the renal and pancreatic lesions. The most common causes of failure of a biphasic spiral CT of the upper abdomen are congestive heart failure or poor cardiac output. These patients are probably best studied by gadolinium-enhanced magnetic resonance imaging (MRI), which is not limited to two acquisitions. Timing is, therefore, not critical, because multiple gradient echo breathshold images can be obtained to optimize enhancement of the pancreas and liver.

References

Dupuy DE, Costello P, Ecker CP. Spiral CT of the pancreas. *Radiology* 1992; 183:815–818.

Eelkema EA, Stephens DH, Ward EM, et al. CT features of nonfunctioning islet cell carcinoma. *AJR* 1984; 143:943–948.

Fishman EK, Wyatt SH, Ney DR, et al. Spiral CT of the pancreas with multiplanar display. *AJR* 1992; 159:1209–1215.

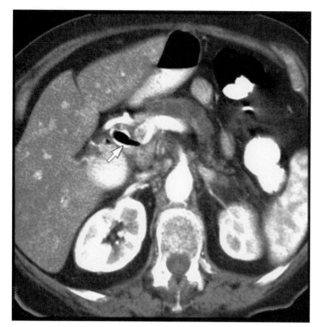

FIG. 136A. CT:arterial phase

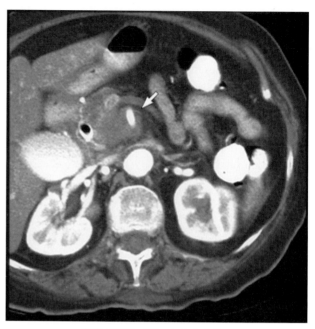

FIG. 136B. CT:arterial phase

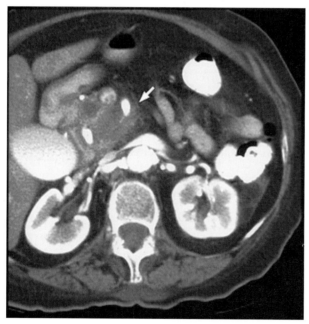

FIG. 136C. CT:arterial phase

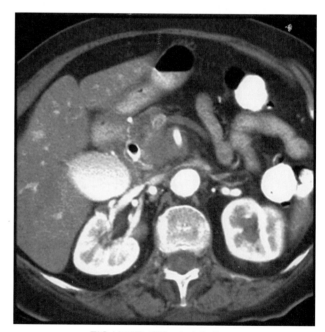

FIG. 136D. CT:arterial phase

History

Obstructive jaundice from pancreatic carcinoma. Determine resectability.

Findings

Figures 136A–D are arterial-phase scans in a biphasic spiral CT study of the pancreas. Notice in Figure 136A that there is distal atrophy of the pancreatic parenchyma, with an enlarged pancreatic duct. Gas is noted within a biliary endoprosthesis (arrow). Note in Figures 136B and C that there is extensive encasement of the origin and root of the superior mesenteric artery (arrow). Figure 136D demonstrates tumor encasement of proximal jejunal branches of the artery.

Diagnosis

Unresectable pancreatic carcinoma with arterial encasement.

Discussion

The use of thin collimation (3 mm) and the rapid-bolus technique affords excellent opacification of the celiac artery and superior mesenteric artery and its branches. Arterial encasement virtually precludes curative surgery in these patients, because there is extrapancreatic extension of the tumor. Even relatively small vessels, such as jejunal branches and inferior pancreatic duodenal arcades, can be readily imaged with current spiral CT technique. CT is highly reliable when there are clear-cut signs of unresectability. Patients with small tumors on CT that appear to be resectable may have positive nodes at surgery that are of normal size on preoperative CT.

References

Nghiem HV, Freeny PC. Radiologic staging of pancreatic adenocarcinoma. *Radiol Clin North Am* 1994; 32:71–79.
Thoeni RF, Blankenberg F. Pancreatic imaging. Computed tomography and magnetic resonance imaging. *Radiol Clin North Am* 1993; 31:1085–1113.

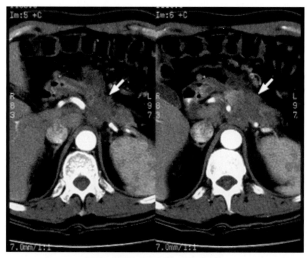

FIG. 137A. CT:arterial phase

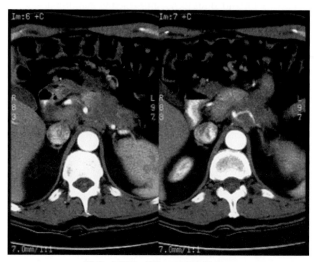

FIG. 137B. CT:arterial phase

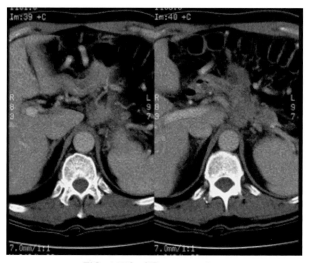

FIG. 137C. CT:venous phase

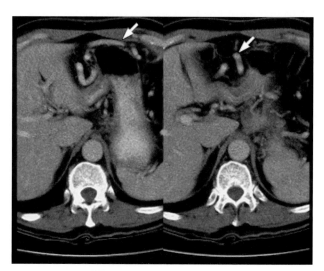

FIG. 137D. CT:venous phase

History

Weight loss and back pain in a 74-year-old male. Rule out pancreatic carcinoma.

Findings

Figures 137A and B are scans obtained during the arterial phase of a biphasic spiral CT study of the pancreas. Note the encasement of the splenic artery by tumor, with direct extension posterior to the pancreas involving the celiac axis (arrows). Figures 137C and D are scans obtained during the portal venous phase. Notice that there is a lack of visualization of the splenic vein in Figure 137C, and the very prominent short gastric and gastroepiploic varices in Figure 137D (arrows).

Diagnosis

Pancreatic carcinoma with splenic vein occlusion and encasement of the splenic artery.

Discussion

This case illustrates the value of combining arterial- and portal-venous-phase images to accurately stage patients with pancreatic carcinoma. The arterial-phase images are best for delineating tumor encasement involving branches of the splanchnic vasculature. The portal-venous phase optimally demonstrates venous occlusion and collateral venous pathways. Patients with splenic-vein occlusion typically demonstrate enlarged, short gastric, gastroepiploic, and splenic-hilus varices. This finding generally indicates a very poor prognosis and generally suggests that the tumor is not resectable for a cure, because there is peripancreatic extension of tumor. Portal-venous-phase images are often most useful in identifying liver metastases.

References

Nghiem HV, Freeny PC. Radiologic staging of pancreatic adenocarcinoma. *Radiol Clin North Am* 1994; 32:71–79.
Thoeni RF, Blankenberg F. Pancreatic imaging. Computed tomography and magnetic resonance imaging. *Radiol Clin North Am* 1993; 31:1085–1113.

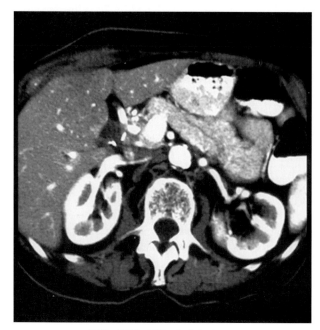

FIG. 138A. CT:arterial phase

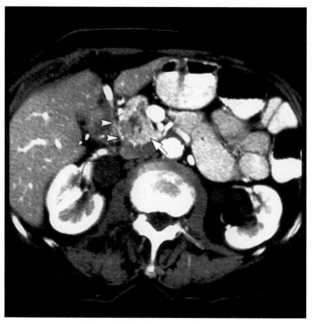

FIG. 138B. CT:arterial phase

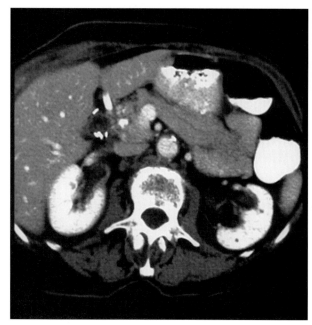

FIG. 138C. CT:venous phase

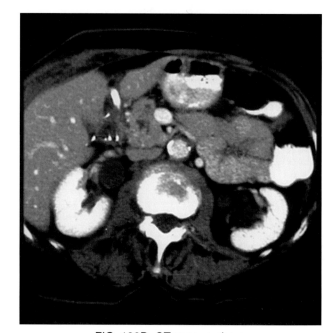

FIG. 138D. CT:venous phase

History

Painless jaundice. Rule out pancreatic carcinoma.

Findings

Figures 138A and B are arterial-phase scans obtained during a biphasic spiral CT study of the pancreas. Note the intense opacification of the normal tail of the pancreas in Figure 138A. A normal size pancreatic duct is well seen in the distal portion of the gland. In Figure 138B, a heterogeneous low-attenuation mass is identified in the head of the pancreas (arrow). The mass does not involve either the superior mesenteric artery or vein. Notice the enhancing vessels on the surface of the pancreas, representing inferior pancreatic duodenal arcades (arrowheads). Figures 138C and D are portal-venous-phase scans at the same corresponding levels demonstrating significantly decreased attenuation of the pancreatic parenchyma. The pancreatic neoplasm in Figure 138D is very difficult to identify, and is seen only as a very small low-attenuation area.

Diagnosis

Pancreatic carcinoma more clearly identified on arterial-phase images.

Discussion

One of the main indications for spiral CT of the pancreas is to stage patients with probable carcinomas in order to determine whether they are potential surgical candidates. In this patient the true extent of the tumor in the head of the pancreas was best delineated on the arterial-phase images. The lack of tumor involvement of surface vascularity on the head of the pancreas suggests that there has not been invasion through the pancreatic capsule.

Although CT cannot distinguish metastasis to normal sized lymph nodes, biphasic spiral CT of the pancreas with thin sections and the rapid bolus technique appears to have significant advantages in identifying vascular encasement. This patient had a successful Whipple resection of the pancreatic carcinoma, without positive lymph nodes.

References

Dupuy DE, Costello P, Ecker CP. Spiral CT of the pancreas. *Radiology* 1992; 183:815–818.

Fishman EK, Wyatt SH, Ney DR, et al. Spiral CT of the pancreas with multiplanar display. *AJR* 1992; 159:1209–1215.

Hollett MD, Jorgensen MJ, Jeffrey RB Jr. Quantitative evaluation of pancreatic enhancement during dual-phase helical CT. *Radiology* 1995; 195:363–370.

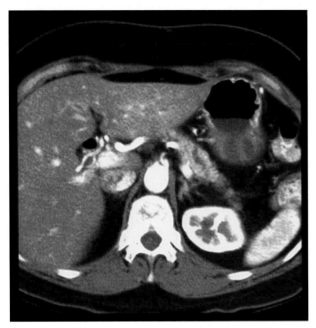

FIG. 139A. CT:arterial phase

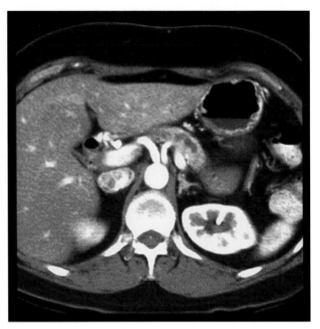

FIG. 139B. CT:arterial phase

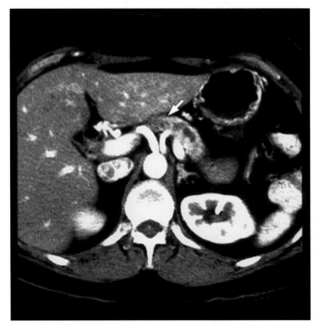

FIG. 139C. CT:arterial phase

History

Vague midepigastric pain. Rule out pancreatic carcinoma.

Findings

Figures 139A–C are arterial-phase images of a biphasic spiral CT study of the pancreas. Note the intense opacification of the pancreatic parenchyma, which is of significantly greater attenuation than the adjacent liver. The pancreatic duct is clearly evident and is dilated. There is excellent opacification of the celiac axis and the splenic artery. In Figure 139C (which is photographed at narrow windows), note the obstruction of the pancreatic duct by a small tumor within the body of the pancreas (arrow). The mass is located adjacent to the bifurcation of the hepatic and splenic arteries.

Diagnosis

Small adenocarcinoma of the pancreas visible on narrow windows.

Discussion

Arterial-phase imaging with a rapid-bolus technique results in intense opacification of the normal pancreas. Conversely, the hepatic parenchyma is often poorly enhanced in these images because it derives 80% of its blood supply from the portal vein. Small hypovascular pancreatic lesions, such as in ductal adenocarcinoma, are often best appreciated in arterial-phase images. In this patient there is an "interrupted duct sign." The small, hypodense tumor is seen immediately adjacent to the dilated pancreatic duct in the tail of the pancreas. It is very important to scrutinize areas of dilatation of the pancreatic duct for small adjacent masses. Any pancreatic neoplasm may result in the "interrupted duct sign," which is not specific for ductal adenocarcinoma. However, given the fact that 80 to 90% of all solid masses in the pancreas are ductal adenocarcinomas, this is far and away the most likely diagnosis. One other technical point to be emphasized with pancreatic imaging is that narrow windows are often very helpful to increase the conspicuity of low-density lesions.

References

Dupuy DE, Costello P, Ecker CP. Spiral CT of the pancreas. *Radiology* 1992; 183:815–818.

Fishman EK, Wyatt SH, Ney DR, et al. Spiral CT of the pancreas with multiplanar display. *AJR* 1992; 159:1209–1215.

Hollett MD, Jorgensen MJ, Jeffrey RB Jr. Quantitative evaluation of pancreatic enhancement during dual-phase helical CT. *Radiology* 1995; 195:363–370.

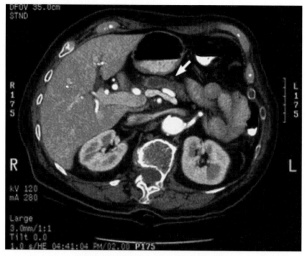

FIG. 140A. CT:arterial phase

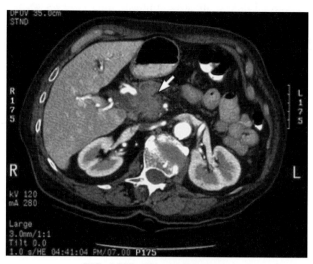

FIG. 140B. CT:arterial phase

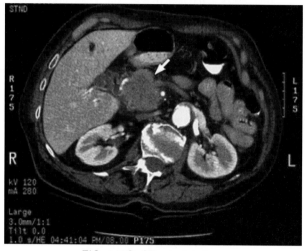

FIG. 140C. CT:arterial phase

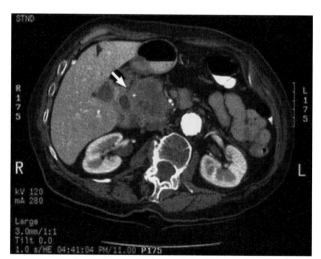

FIG. 140D. CT:arterial phase

History

Back pain in a 79-year-old female. Rule out pancreatic carcinoma.

Findings

Figures 140A–D are arterial-phase images of the pancreas obtained during a biphasic spiral CT scan. Note in Figure 140A the distal atrophy of the pancreas and the dilated pancreatic duct (arrow). Figures 140B and C demonstrate a large mass arising from the head of the pancreas (arrow) and extending into the porta hepatis, encasing the hepatic artery. Note the excellent opacification of the hepatic artery during the arterial-phase images. Figure 140D demonstrates that the mass encases the gastroduodenal artery (arrow).

Diagnosis

Pancreatic carcinoma encasing the hepatic and gastroduodenal arteries.

Discussion

The extensive hepatic arterial encasement by this pancreatic carcinoma is well demonstrated in the arterial-phase images. This degree of invasion along the hepatic artery makes the tumor not resectable for cure. Arterial encasement is highly characteristic of ductal adenocarcinoma. Other pancreatic neoplasms, such as neuroendocrine tumors, lymphoma, and metastasis rarely produce the same degree of arterial encasement. Venous occlusion, however, can be caused by any of these lesions.

References

Dupuy DE, Costello P, Ecker CP. Spiral CT of the pancreas. *Radiology* 1992; 183:815–818.
Fishman EK, Wyatt SH, Ney DR, et al. Spiral CT of the pancreas with multiplanar display. *AJR* 1992; 159:1209–1215.

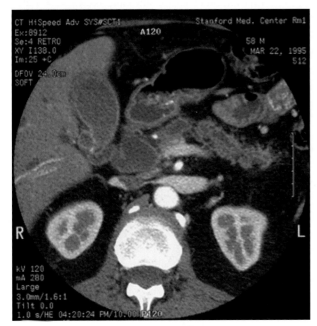

FIG. 141A. CT:arterial phase

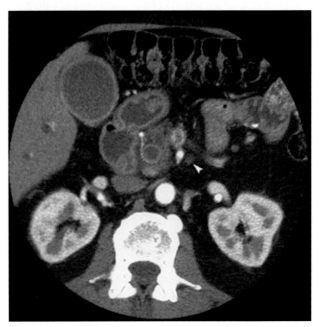

FIG. 141B. CT:arterial phase

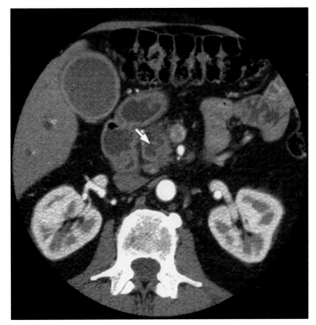

FIG. 141C. CT:arterial phase

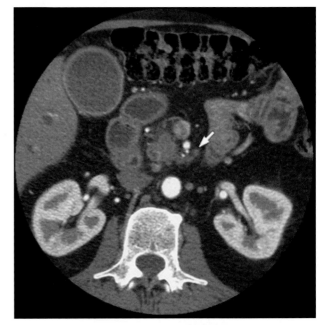

FIG. 141D. CT:arterial phase

History

Painless jaundice. Rule out pancreatic carcinoma.

Findings

Figures 141A–D are arterial-phase scans obtained during a biphasic spiral CT study of the pancreas. Notice in Figure 141A the "double duct sign," with dilatation of both the common bile duct and the pancreatic duct. In Figure 141B there is excellent opacification of the mucosa of the common bile duct. Notice the small nodes adjacent to the superior mesenteric artery in Figures 141A and B (arrowhead). In Figure 141C the ring enhancement of the mucosa of the common bile duct is interrupted by tumor (arrow), which obstructs the pancreatic and common bile ducts at this level. In Figure 141D the low-attenuation tumor has extended posteriorly to the superior mesenteric artery near the root of the mesentery (arrow).

Diagnosis

Pancreatic carcinoma with metastatic lymphadenopathy involving the root of the mesentery.

Discussion

The rapid-bolus spiral CT scan in this patient identified the enhancing normal mucosa of the common bile duct as well as the site of tumor infiltration. In addition, the lymphadenopathy involving the root of the mesentery was clearly identified posterior to the superior mesenteric artery. At surgery, four of nine peripancreatic lymph nodes were positive for tumor. Postoperatively the patient developed extensive chylous ascites from lymphatic leakage. This resolved spontaneously after 1 week.

References

Nghiem HV, Freeny PC. Radiologic staging of pancreatic adenocarcinoma. *Radiol Clin North Am* 1994; 32:71–79.
Thoeni RF, Blankenberg F. Pancreatic imaging. Computed tomography and magnetic resonance imaging. *Radiol Clin North Am* 1993; 31:1085–1113.

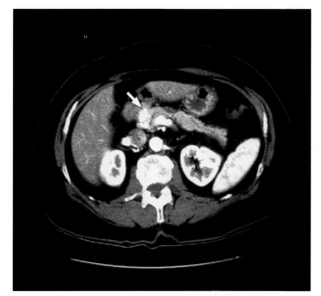

FIG. 142A. CT:arterial phase

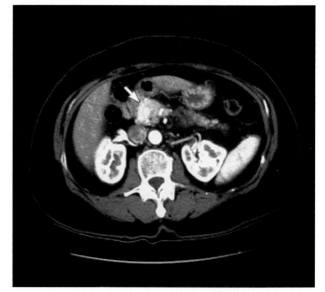

FIG. 142B. CT:arterial phase

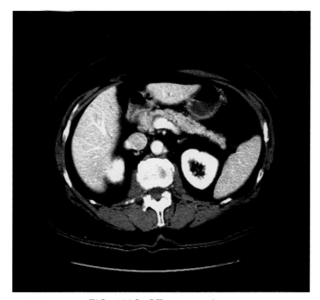

FIG. 142C. CT:venous phase

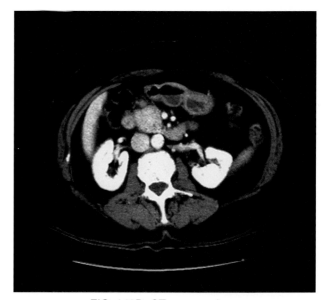

FIG. 142D. CT:venous phase

History

A 64-year-old female with vague midepigastric pain. Sonography suggests a possible mass in the head of the pancreas.

Findings

Figures 142A and B are early arterial-phase images from a dual-phase spiral CT study of the pancreas. Note the hypervascular mass involving the head and neck of the pancreas (arrow). Figures 142C and D are scans through the pancreas obtained during the portal venous phase, demonstrating a vague mass effect in the region of the head of the pancreas, without delineation of a discrete lesion.

Diagnosis

Neuroendocrine tumor of the pancreas.

Discussion

Rapid-bolus, dual-phase imaging of the pancreas affords a number of important diagnostic advantages. Arterial encasement by tumor is clearly demonstrated, as well as increased conspicuity of both hypo- and hypervascular parenchymal masses within the pancreas. Ductal adenocarcinoma accounts for 80 to 90% of all solid pancreatic masses. It is typically a hypovascular lesion and thus would not be expected to demonstrate increased vascularity as compared to the normal pancreas. Given the hypervascular nature of the mass in this patient, the most likely diagnosis is a neuroendocrine tumor of the pancreas. Rarely, hypervascular metastasis to the pancreas from renal-cell carcinoma or melanoma may occur and should be included in the differential diagnosis. Neuroendocrine tumors (islet-cell neoplasms) may be either functioning or nonfunctioning. Nonfunctioning neuroendocrine tumors are often quite bulky in size, typically measuring 6 to 10 cm in diameter.

Of particular note in this case is that the neuroendocrine tumor is poorly visualized during the portal venous phase, because it is nearly isodense with the remainder of the pancreas. The increased vascularity of the lesion is only appreciated in the arterial-phase images. The arterial-phase images are generally acquired after a 25-second scan delay. An arterial-phase spiral CT acquisition through the pancreas is best performed with a collimation of 3 to 5 mm in order not to miss small lesions. Following rebreathing and repositioning of the patient, portal-venous-phase scans are done through the liver and kidneys in order to detect liver metastasis and venous obstruction.

References

Eelkema EA, Stephens DH, Ward EM, et al. CT features of nonfunctioning islet cell carcinoma. *AJR* 1984; 143:943–948.

Fishman EK, Wyatt SH, Ney DR, et al. Spiral CT of the pancreas with multiplanar display. *AJR* 1992; 159:1209–1215.

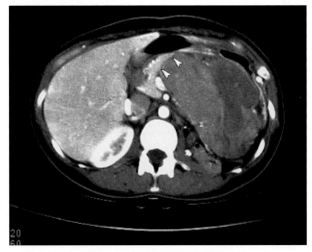

FIG. 143A. CT:arterial phase

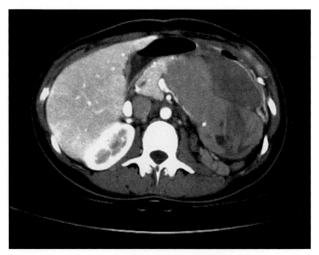

FIG. 143B. CT:arterial phase

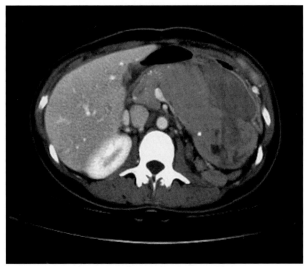

FIG. 143C. CT:venous phase

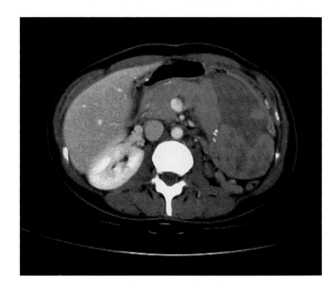

FIG. 143D. CT:venous phase

History

This patient had undergone resection of liposarcoma of the left upper quadrant with splenectomy, distal pancreatectomy, and nephrectomy. The patient has an enlarging abdominal mass.

Findings

Figures 143A and B are arterial-phase images from a biphasic spiral CT study of the abdomen. Note the sharp demarcation between the normal pancreatic parenchyma (arrowheads) and the large heterogeneous mass in the left upper quadrant. Figures 143C and D are scans obtained during the portal venous phase. A small amount of fat is noted in the mass posteriorly. Notice that the interface with the normal pancreas is poorly identified, and that invasion of the pancreas cannot clearly be determined with these images.

Diagnosis

Recurrent liposarcoma extrinsically compressing the pancreas.

Discussion

The arterial-phase images in this patient clearly revealed a sharp interface between the recurrent tumor and the normally enhancing pancreas. Based on the arterial-phase images, it is clear that the tumor extrinsically compresses the pancreas rather than directly invading it. This, however, is not clearly evident on the portal-venous-phase images, since there is no sharp demarcation between the mass and the pancreas. At surgery there was an extrinsic mass effect on the pancreas, without evidence of invasion.

References

Ferrozzi F, Bova D, Garlaschi G. Gastric liposarcoma: CT appearance. *Abdom Imag* 1993; 18:232–233.
Springfield D. Liposarcoma. *Clin Orthopaed Rel Res* 1993; 289:50–57.

The Retroperitoneum

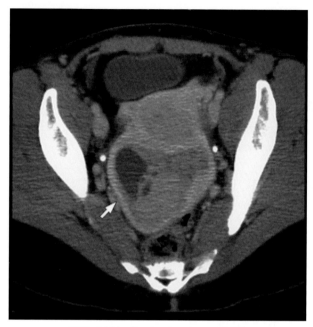

FIG. 144A. Contrast-enhanced CT

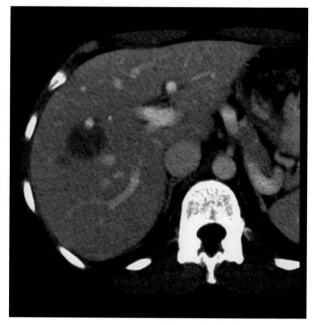

FIG. 144B. Contrast-enhanced CT

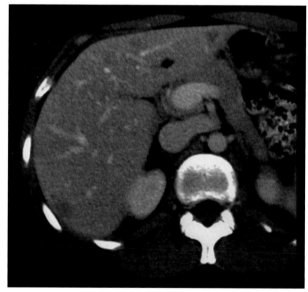

FIG. 144C. Contrast-enhanced CT

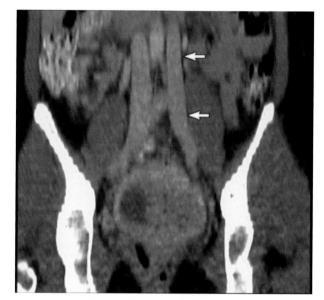

FIG. 144D. Coronal reformation

History

Enlarging uterus and increased liver function test valves.

Findings

Figures 144A–C are axial scans obtained from a contrast-enhanced spiral CT study of the abdomen and pelvis. Note the large heterogeneous mass involving the uterus in Figure 144A (arrow). Figures 144B and C demonstrate multiple focal hepatic lesions. Figure 144D is a coronal reformation of the pelvis demonstrating a duplicated inferior vena cava (arrows) displaced by the large pelvic mass.

Diagnosis

Leiomyosarcoma of the uterus, hepatic metastasis, and duplication of the inferior vena cava.

Discussion

The heterogeneous uterine mass in this patient at surgery proved to be a leiomyosarcoma. Unfortunately, at the time of presentation, multiple liver metastases were diagnosed with CT. The coronal reformations were helpful for avoiding vascular injury at surgery, because they made the surgeons aware of the duplicated inferior vena cava. Excellent contrast enhancement of the upper abdomen and pelvis afforded by the spiral CT facilitated multiplanar reformations. The coronal plane clearly demonstrates the duplicated inferior vena cava. Duplication of the inferior vena cava has a prevalence of 0.2 to 3%. The left-sided inferior vena cava usually enters the left renal vein.

References

Gomes MN, Choyke PL. Assessment of major venous anomalies by computerized tomography. *J Cardiovasc Surg* 1990; 31:621–628.

Levine E. "The retroperitoneum." In: Putman CE, Ravin CE (eds.): *Textbook of Diagnostic Imaging*, 2nd ed. Philadelphia: WB Saunders, 1994, pp. 1209.

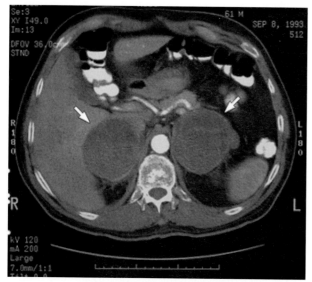

FIG. 145A. CT:arterial phase

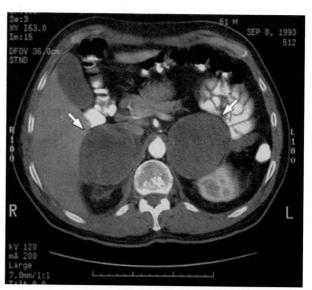

FIG. 145B. CT:arterial phase]

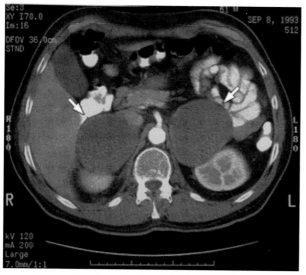

FIG. 145C. CT:arterial phase

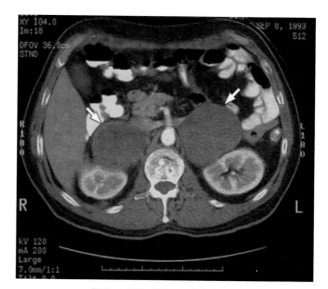

FIG. 145D. CT:arterial phase

History

A 61-year-old man with melanoma and back pain.

Findings

Figures 145A–D are arterial-phase images from a biphasic spiral CT study of the upper abdomen. Note on all four images the large, low-attenuating adrenal lesions without significant enhancement (arrows).

Diagnosis

Bilateral necrotic adrenal metastasis from melanoma.

Discussion

The large bilateral adrenal masses in this case were due to metastases from melanoma. The lack of significant arterial-phase enhancement is consistent with necrosis, which was proven at autopsy. Although granulomatous infection, pheochromocytomas, and other benign adrenal disorders such as hemorrhage may occur bilaterally, the marked distortion of the normal adrenal morphology and the rounded nature of the lesion in this case strongly favors metastasis. Melanoma may produce hypervascular metastases. However, when significant hemorrhage and necrosis occur, the lesions will not demonstrate significant enhancement with spiral CT. CT is an excellent method for guiding the percutaneous biopsy of suspected adrenal metastases.

References

Branum GD, Epstein RE, Leight GS, Seigler HF. The role of resection in the management of melanoma metastatic to the adrenal gland. *Surgery* 1991; 109:127–131.

Khafagi FA, Gross MD, Shapiro B, Glazer GM, Francis I, Thompson NW. Clinical significance of the large adrenal mass. *Br J Surgery* 1991; 73:828–833.

Singer AA, Obuchowski NA, Einstein DM, Paushter DM. Metastasis or adenoma? Computed tomographic evaluation of the adrenal mass. *Cleve Clin J Med* 1994; 61:200–205.

Tikkakoski T, Taavitsainen M, Paivansalo M, Lahde S, Apaja-Sarkkinen M. Accuracy of adrenal biopsy guided by ultrasound and CT. *Acta Radiol* 1991; 32:371–374.

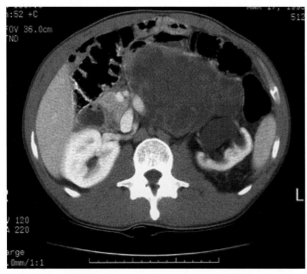

FIG. 146A. Contrast-enhanced CT

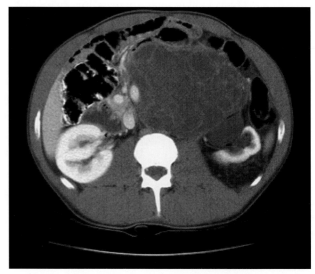

FIG. 146B. Contrast-enhanced CT

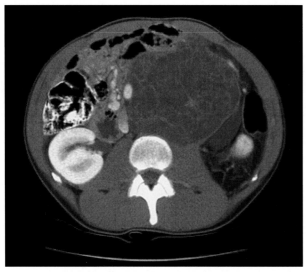

FIG. 146C. Contrast-enhanced CT

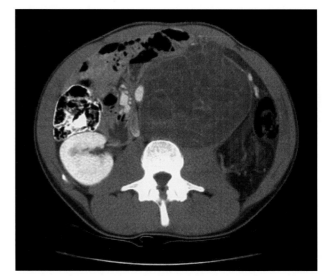

FIG. 146D. Contrast-enhanced CT

History

This patient had undergone resection of left testicular carcinoma, and now had an increasing abdominal girth.

Findings

Figures 146A–D are contrast-enhanced spiral CT images of the midabdomen, demonstrating a large cystic mass displacing the aorta and inferior vena cava anteriorly and to the right. The mass is predominantly cystic, with enhancing internal septa.

Diagnosis

Recurrent testicular carcinoma metastatic to the retroperitoneum.

Discussion

The excellent contrast enhancement of the spiral CT images in this case clearly demonstrated the enhancing septa within the patient's cystic mass, representing metastatic testicular carcinoma. Surgery revealed teratocarcinoma with myxoid elements. One of the advantages of spiral CT is more reliable contrast enhancement. Thus, smaller blood vessels can be more consistently imaged.

Fat-containing retroperitoneal metastases in teratocarcinoma may in fact represent benign teratomas. Benign teratomas may develop in the retroperitoneum in patients with prior nodal metastases. Not infrequently, these teratomas may be quite large, on the order of 5 to 8 cm. A small percentage of these lesions will contain foci of carcinoma and, hence, are generally surgically resected.

References

Coscojuela P, Llauger J, Perez C, Germa J, Castaner B. The growing teratoma syndrome: radiologic findings in four cases. *Eur J Radiol* 1991; 12:138–140.

Saganlowsky AI, Ewalt DH, Molberg K, Peters PC. Predictors of residual mass histology after chemotherapy for advanced testis cancer. *Urology* 1990; 35:537–542.

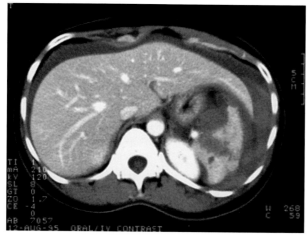

FIG. 147A. Contrast-enhanced CT

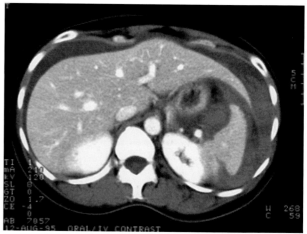

FIG. 147B. Contrast-enhanced CT

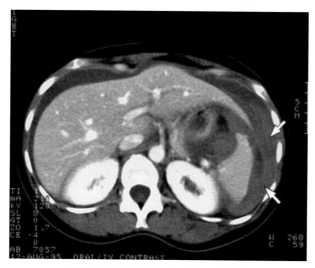

FIG. 147C. Contrast-enhanced CT

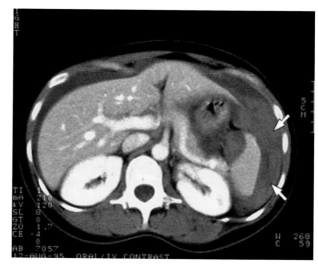

FIG. 147D. Contrast-enhanced CT

History

A 34-year-old female who was involved in a motor-vehicle accident approximately 1 week before admission, with a known left rib fracture. The patient was originally seen at a hospital emergency room and discharged. She developed nausea and dizziness with left-upper-quadrant pain and returned to the emergency room. A spiral CT of the abdomen was obtained.

314

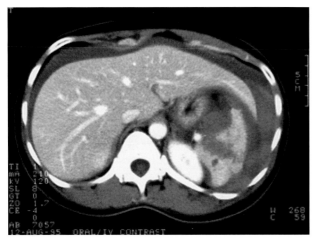

FIG. 147A. Contrast-enhanced CT

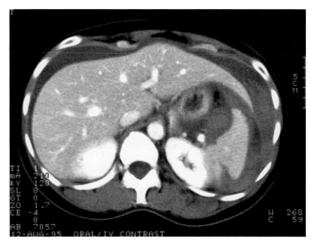

FIG. 147B. Contrast-enhanced CT

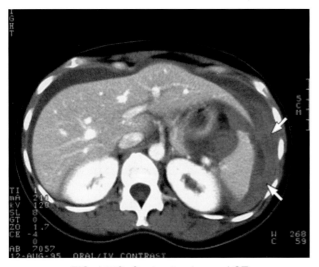

FIG. 147C. Contrast-enhanced CT

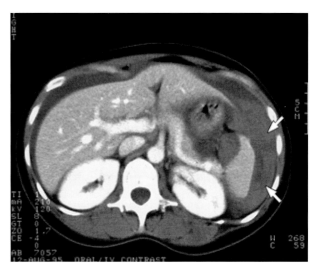

FIG. 147D. Contrast-enhanced CT

History

A 34-year-old female who was involved in a motor-vehicle accident approximately 1 week before admission, with a known left rib fracture. The patient was originally seen at a hospital emergency room and discharged. She developed nausea and dizziness with left-upper-quadrant pain and returned to the emergency room. A spiral CT of the abdomen was obtained.

314

SECTION 11

The Spleen

Findings

Figures 146A–D are contrast-enhanced spiral CT images of the midabdomen, demonstrating a large cystic mass displacing the aorta and inferior vena cava anteriorly and to the right. The mass is predominantly cystic, with enhancing internal septa.

Diagnosis

Recurrent testicular carcinoma metastatic to the retroperitoneum.

Discussion

The excellent contrast enhancement of the spiral CT images in this case clearly demonstrated the enhancing septa within the patient's cystic mass, representing metastatic testicular carcinoma. Surgery revealed teratocarcinoma with myxoid elements. One of the advantages of spiral CT is more reliable contrast enhancement. Thus, smaller blood vessels can be more consistently imaged.

Fat-containing retroperitoneal metastases in teratocarcinoma may in fact represent benign teratomas. Benign teratomas may develop in the retroperitoneum in patients with prior nodal metastases. Not infrequently, these teratomas may be quite large, on the order of 5 to 8 cm. A small percentage of these lesions will contain foci of carcinoma and, hence, are generally surgically resected.

References

Coscojuela P, Llauger J, Perez C, Germa J, Castaner B. The growing teratoma syndrome: radiologic findings in four cases. *Eur J Radiol* 1991; 12:138–140.

Saganlowsky AI, Ewalt DH, Molberg K, Peters PC. Predictors of residual mass histology after chemotherapy for advanced testis cancer. *Urology* 1990; 35:537–542.

Findings

The spiral CT scan demonstrates a laceration through the hilum of the spleen, with evidence of hemoperitoneum. The blood is densest around the spleen and left lower lobe of the liver, which is consistent with a sentinel clot sign.

Diagnosis

Delayed splenic rupture with hemoperitoneum.

Discussion

Spiral CT has important benefits in the evaluation of patient status following trauma. The known benefits of CT are amplified with spiral CT, which requires less time for completion: a factor that is often critical in the traumatized or semistable patient. A spiral CT scan of the abdomen can be done as a single scan in 24 to 40 seconds. The fast scanning is important in minimizing motion artifacts in trauma patients, who may have difficulty in cooperating for the standard study, which takes between 5 and 15 minutes. The ability to obtain data sets during peak intravenous contrast enhancement is particularly valuable in detecting injuries to the liver or spleen. Specific problems with irregular splenic enhancement, which are described in the arterial phase, are not problematic if scanning is done around 60 to 70 seconds after injection of contrast medium.

Delayed splenic rupture is a well-known entity. Since many patients with abdominal trauma are managed conservatively without imaging, it is not surprising that a splenic injury can be fairly significant yet self-contained, and might therefore be overlooked. These patients typically present several days later if additional bleeding occurs or if the spleen ruptures. Since many patients with CT scans and splenic injury are followed conservatively, it would not be surprising to see an increased incidence of delayed splenic rupture.

The role of follow-up CT scans in the patient with splenic injury is a topic of some controversy. It is important to recognize that the radiologist must be aware of the possibility of delayed splenic rupture in patients with a prior history of trauma and severe abdominal pain, particularly if the latter is localized to the left or right upper quadrant. In these cases, CT is an ideal study for excluding this possibility.

References

Bundy AL, Scott M, Druckman D, Siegal TL, Verdi TA. Delayed and occult splenic rupture. *Computer Radiol* 1985; 9:299–305.

Pretorius ES, Fishman EK. Spiral computed tomography of upper abdominal trauma. *Emer Radiol* 1995; 2:285–289.

Taylor AJ, Dodds WJ, Erickson SJ, Stewart ET. CT of acquired abnormalities of the spleen. *AJR* 1991; 157:1213–1219.

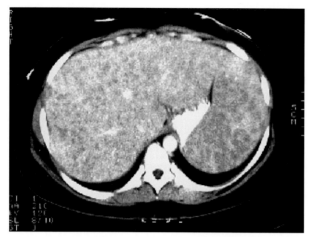

FIG. 148A. Contrast-enhanced CT

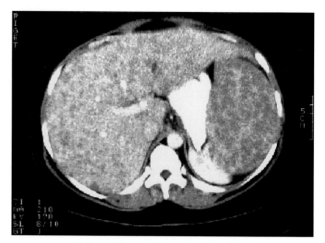

FIG. 148B. Contrast-enhanced CT

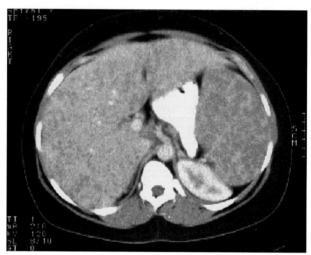

FIG. 148C. Contrast-enhanced CT

History

A 27-year-old black female with a history of neurosarcoidosis and recent onset of dysphagia and abdominal pain. The patient also had elevated liver function tests.

Findings

A spiral CT scan demonstrates moderate hepatosplenomegaly. Multiple low-density lesions are seen throughout both the liver and spleen. The lesions demonstrate no evidence of enhancement. No evidence of calcification was present. The differential diagnosis would include infiltrating processes of the liver and spleen, including malignancies (lymphoma or metastases) and infectious processes (fungal infection, cat-scratch fever, or sarcoidosis).

Diagnosis

Sarcoidosis of the liver and spleen.

Discussion

Warshauer recently reported a series of 32 cases of nodular hepatosplenic sarcoidosis that were gathered from the files of seven major medical institutions. In general, sarcoidosis can involve the liver or spleen, although involvement on radiographic imaging studies has been infrequent. In part, this is due to the infiltrating nature of the disease process. Needle biopsy of the spleen in an unselected population of patients with sarcoid will demonstrate involvement in up to 59% of cases. In cases in which CT scans are positive, this is most commonly due to hepatosplenomegaly. In other cases, sarcoidosis can manifest as multiple low-attenuation nodules that can be confused with either malignancy or infectious etiologies. In the Warshauer series of 32 patients with nodular hepatosplenic sarcoidosis, the nodules were particularly small, multiple, and of low CT attenuation. Abdominal adenopathy was present in 76% of these patients, and up to one-quarter of the patients had normal chest radiographs.

It is important to recognize abdominal manifestations of sarcoidosis, whether they involve the liver, spleen, or lymph nodes. It is important to remember this because the process can easily be confused with a malignancy. Britt et al. previously compared the CT findings in 16 patients with abdominal sarcoidosis with those in 20 patients with non-Hodgkin lymphoma and noted that the two diseases could look very similar. In that article, retrocrural adenopathy was one of the key differentiating factors, and was far less common in sarcoidosis than in lymphoma. With spiral CT now being used on a routine basis, more cases of infiltration of the spleen and liver by inflammatory and infectious processes will be discovered. It is important to recognize that sarcoidosis can cause this pattern, and in the patient with sarcoidosis, infiltration of the liver and spleen should be considered presumptive of abdominal sarcoid rather than as indicating a metastatic neoplasm or lymphoma.

References

Britt AR, Francis IR, Glazer GM, Ellis JH. Sarcoidosis: abdominal manifestations at CT. *Radiology* 1991; 178:91–94.

Warshauer DM, Dumbleton SA, Molina PL, Yankaskas BC, Parker LA, Woosley JT. Abdominal CT findings in sarcoidosis: radiologic and clinical correlation. *Radiology* 1994; 192:93–98.

Warshauer DM, Molina PL, Hamman SM, et al. Nodular sarcoidosis of the liver and spleen: analysis of 32 cases. *Radiology* 1995; 195:757–762.

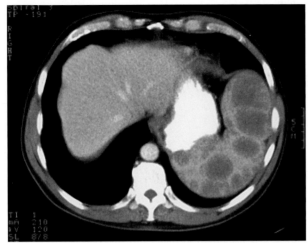

FIG. 149A. Contrast-enhanced CT

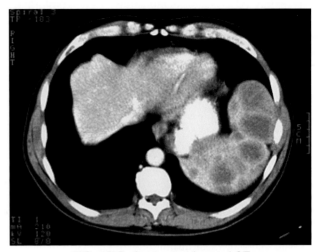

FIG. 149B. Contrast-enhanced CT

History

A 62-year-old male with a history of abdominal pain. No other history was available at the time of the study.

Findings

A spiral CT scan demonstrates an enlarged spleen with multiple solid lesions within the splenic parenchyma. The lesions measure between 1 and 5 cm in size. No associated adenopathy or hepatic lesions were seen.

Diagnosis

Gaucher disease of the spleen.

Discussion

Spiral CT provides a potential opportunity for improving the accuracy of evaluation of splenic pathology. Although there has been no formal study to date, it has been our impression that with spiral CT, it is substantially easier to detect lesions, whether they are diffuse or more focal. Although there is the potential for pseudolesions in early-phase images, this is usually not too much of a clinical problem, since the appearance (commonly a moiré pattern) tends to be easily recognized with experience.

One limitation of spiral CT is that at times it is very sensitive for the detection of disease but not very specific as to the exact diagnosis. In the present case, the spleen is enlarged, with multiple low-density lesions. Considering the patient's age and history, the differential diagnosis would be extensive, but would suggest malignancy such as lymphoma or metastatic disease (such as melanoma or lung cancer). The possibility of benign tumor nodules such as hemangiomas would also be a consideration, although it would be less likely because of the size of the spleen. Other possibilities, such as infection or infarction, are also considerations. However, infarction is unlikely, considering that the lesions are fairly round. Although infection is also unlikely, it cannot be fully excluded on the basis only of the CT appearance.

The patient had a bone-marrow biopsy, and the diagnosis was Gaucher disease.

Gaucher disease is an unusual hereditary lysosomal storage disease. There are three forms of the disease: the infantile, juvenile, and adult forms. The adult form is probably the most common of all lysosomal storage diseases. As in the present case, the patient usually presents with splenomegaly or thrombocytopenia. Other complications typically involve the skeletal system, and include pathologic fractures, vertebral-body collapse, and avascular necrosis of the femoral heads.

Gaucher disease has rarely been reported in the radiologic literature, particularly with CT imaging. A few reported cases have shown multiple low-density lesions in the spleen without any evidence of other organ involvement. There have been several reports of the ultrasound findings of multiple hypo- or hyperechoic lesions.

The patient with Gaucher disease can have a variable course, and some patients have a normal life span while others develop pulmonary involvement or hepatic failure resulting in early demise.

References

Aspestrand F, Charania B, Scheel B, et al. Focal changes of the spleen in one case of Gaucher's disease assessed by ultrasonography, CT, MRI, and angiography. *Radiology* 1989; 29:569–571.

Hill SC, Reinig JW, Barranger JA, et al. Gaucher's disease: sonographic appearance of the spleen. *Radiology* 1986; 160:631–634.

Tupler RH, Trent CC, McDonald KL. Radiological case of the month. *Appl Radiol* 1991; 20:30–31.

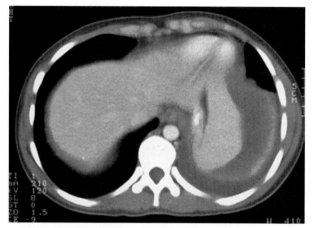

FIG. 150A. Contrast-enhanced CT

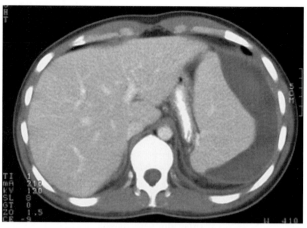

FIG. 150B. Contrast-enhanced CT

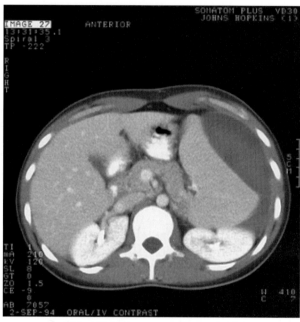

FIG. 150C. Contrast-enhanced CT

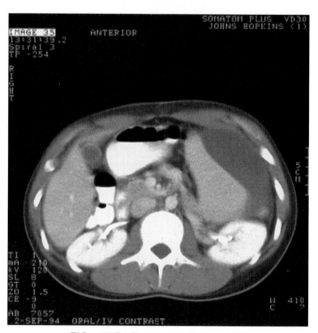

FIG. 150D. Contrast-enhanced CT

History

A 20-year-old male with a history of infectious mononucleosis and increasing left-upper-quadrant pain.

Findings

Spiral CT scan demonstrates a large subcapsular collection involving the lateral portion of the spleen. The fluid is of high CT attenuation. The patient has no history of recent trauma or any other clinical history besides the diagnosis of infectious mononucleosis.

Diagnosis

Subcapsular hematoma of the spleen.

Discussion

Imaging the spleen has always been one of the great challenges in diagnostic radiology. Whether the modality is CT, magnetic resonance imaging (MRI), ultrasound, or nuclear medicine, there have always been substantial limitations in the detection of splenic pathology. Spiral CT scanning has proven very useful in evaluation of the spleen, and in our experience has been sensitive to infiltrating processes as well as small tumor masses in the spleen. One pitfall of spiral CT is that when the spleen is scanned early, particularly at about 30 to 40 seconds after the injection of contrast medium is initiated, the splenic enhancement due to the organ's blood supply will be irregular and is often seen as a Moiré-type pattern. In this phase it may be difficult to distinguish between an infiltrating process and normal irregular enhancement.

For complications of splenic injury, including splenic laceration and hemorrhage, spiral CT accentuates both the normal and abnormal tissue, making detection of subtle lesions apparent. In the present case, the CT study clearly demonstrates the large subcapsular collection compressing normal splenic tissue. No evidence of a splenic laceration is seen. The fluid is of high CT attenuation, consistent with blood. Spiral CT has been previously shown to be very accurate in the definition of attenuation values. The diagnosis in this case is therefore spontaneous subcapsular hematoma in a patient with infectious mononucleosis. Because of the clinical history, the patient was managed conservatively and no intervention was planned unless further symptoms developed. It should be noted that in patients with infectious mononucleosis, spontaneous splenic rupture and hemorrhage are reported in the literature, and that in such cases, careful surveillance of the patient is mandatory.

References

Bundy AL, Scott M, Druckman D, Siegal TL, Verdi TA. Delayed and occult splenic rupture. *Comput Radiol* 1985; 9:299–305.

Rabuska LS, Kawashima A, Fishman EK. Imaging of the spleen: CT with supplemental MR examination. *RadioGraphics* 1994; 14:307–332.

Taylor AJ, Dodds WJ, Erickson SJ, Stewart ET. CT of acquired abnormalities of the spleen. *AJR* 1991; 157:1213–1219.

A

Abdomen, post-traumatic, hemorrhage in, 146–147

Abdominal aorta
aneurysm of, 12–13, 36–37
endoluminal stent graft of, 18–21
ruptured ulcer of, 22–23

Abscess
hepatic, 150–151
renal, 190–191
postpartum, 198–199

Achalasia, 134–135

Acquired immunodeficiency syndrome (AIDS)
anaplastic carcinoma in, 110–111
esophagitis in, 156–157
histoplasmosis in, 193
osteomyelitis in, 268–269
perirectal abscess in, 140–141

Adenocarcinoma
cecal, 152–153
gastric, 180–181
metastatic, 246–247
pancreatic, 294–295
pulmonary, 74–75, 84–85, 94–95

Adenoma, microcystic, pancreatic, 282 283

Adrenal gland
hemorrhage of, 204–205
histoplasmosis of, 192–193
lymphangioma of, 202–203
metastases of, 308–309
myelolipoma of, 203

Anaplastic carcinoma, pulmonary, 110–111

Aneurysm
aortic
abdominal, 12–13, 36–37
endoluminal stent graft of, 18–21
thoracic, 10–14, 28–29, 34–35, 44–45
endoluminal stent graft of, 24–25
mycotic
of hepatic artery, 256–257
of pulmonary artery, 62–63
of thoracic aorta, 10–11

Anticoagulation
adrenal hemorrhage with, 204–205
iliac artery hemorrhage with, 32–33
retroperitoneal hemorrhage with, 26–27

Aorta
abdominal
aneurysm of, 12–13, 36–37
endoluminal stent graft of, 18–21
ruptured ulcer of, 22–23
thoracic
aneurysm of, 28–29, 34–35, 44–45
endoluminal stent graft of, 24–25
dissection of, 28–29, 52–53
mycotic aneurysm of, 10–11
rupture of, 46–47
thoracoabdominal, dissection of, 40–41

Aortic dissection
thoracic, 28–29, 52–53
thoracoabdominal, 40–41

Aortobifemoral graft, 48–49
occlusion of, 50–51

Appendicitis, 128–129, 160–161

Arteriovenous malformation, 38–39

Arteriovenous shunting, in intrahepatic cholangiocarcinoma, 248–249

Ascites, 180–181

Atrial myxoma, 4–5

B

Bacterial endocarditis
hepatic artery aneurysm with, 256–257
pulmonary artery aneurysm with, 62–63

Bile leak, 124–125

Bladder carcinoma, skeletal metastases from, 266–267

Bone, metastases to, from bladder carcinoma, 266–267

Breast carcinoma
chemotherapy for, nodular regenerative hepatic hyperplasia after, 224–225
hepatic metastases from, 230–231
pulmonary metastases from, 116–117

C

Calculus, ureteral, 172–173, 182–183

Candida, in esophagitis, 156–157

Carcinoid tumor, of small bowel, 244–245

Castleman's disease, 86–87

Catheter breakage, in pulmonary artery, 42–43

Cavernous hemangioma, hepatic, 236–237

Cecum
adenocarcinoma of, 152–153
carcinoma of, 200–201

Chemotherapy, nodular regenerative hepatic hyperplasia after, 224–225

Chest wall
anaplastic carcinoma of, 110–111
neoplastic invasion of, 74–75
spindle-cell sarcoma of, 78–79

Child, neuroblastoma in, 108–109, 186–187

Cholangiocarcinoma, 248–249

Cholecystectomy, laparoscopic, complications of, 124–125

Cholecystitis, 122–123

Clear-cell carcinoma, 188–189

Clostridium difficile, colitis, 149

Colitis, pseudomembranous, 148–149

Colon
carcinoma of, 144–145, 152–153, 200–201
gastrocolic fistula with, 158–159
hepatic metastases from, 240–241
metastatic, 162–163, 228–229

sigmoid
Crohn's disease of, 150–151
perforation of, 148–149

Congenital cystic adenomatoid malformation, 82–83

Crohn's disease
of sigmoid colon, 150–151
small-bowel obstruction in, 154–155

Cystadenoma, pancreatic, 276–277

Cystic adenomatoid malformation, 82–83

D

Deltoid muscle, metastatic carcinoma of, 260–261

Double duct sign, 296–299

Duodenum, perforation of, 222–223

E

Embolism, pulmonary, 100–101

Empyema, 80–81, 114–115

Endocarditis, bacterial
hepatic artery aneurysm with, 256–257
pulmonary artery aneurysm with, 62–63

Endoluminal stent graft
of abdominal aortic aneurysm, 18–21
of thoracic aorta rupture, 46–47
of thoracic aortic aneurysm, 24–25, 34–35

Endometriosis, rupture of, 175

Endoscopic retrograde cholangiopancreatography with sphincterotomy, duodenal perforation with, 222–223

Enterolith, 154–155

Enterovaginal fistulae, 178–179

Escherichia coli, in renal abscess, 190–191

Esophagitis, 156–157

Esophagus
achalasia of, 134–135
cancer of, laser therapy of, 168–169
inflammation of, 156–157
perforation of, 168–169

Extralobar sequestration, 60–61

F

Fat
within teratoma, 70–71
thoracic, 68–69

Fistula
enterovaginal, 178–179
gastrocolic, colon carcinoma and, 158–159

Follicular-cell lymphoma, mixed, 196–197

Fracture, sternal, 112–113

G

Gangrene, pulmonary, 118–119

Gas-containing appendix, 160–161

Gastric ulcer, perforation of, 132–133

Gastritis, 164–165
radiation, 138–139

Gastrocolic fistula, colon carcinoma and, 158–159
Gastroduodenal artery, tumor encasement of, 296–297
Gaucher disease, 318–319
Gluteal pseudoaneurysm, 6–7
Gossypibomas, 104–105

H

Heart
  myxoma of, 4–5
  thrombus of, 16–17
  tumors of, 4–5, 17
    metastatic, 30–31
Helicobacter pylori gastritis, 164–165
Hemangioendothelioma, vs. hepatoblastoma, 221
Hemangioma, cavernous, 236–237
Hematoma
  of mediastinum, 112–113
  of spleen, 320–321
Hemorrhage
  abdominal, 146–147
  adrenal, 204–205
  from iliac artery, 32–33
  from lumbar artery, 26–27
  post-traumatic, 146–147
  pulmonary, 118–119
  renal, 206–207
Hepatic artery
  mycotic aneurysm of, 256–257
  tumor encasement of, 296–297
Hepatic vein, cholangiocarcinoma of, 248–249
Hepatoblastoma, 220–221
Hepatocellular carcinoma, 242–243
  atrial extension of, 30–31
  multifocal, 238–239, 252–253
  portal-vein invasion of, 218–219
  recurrence of, 226–227, 234–235
Hepatoma, 30–31
Histoplasmosis, 192–193
Hodgkin disease, 64–65
  spinal, 262–263
Human immunodeficiency virus (HIV), infection with
  anaplastic carcinoma in, 110–111
  esophagitis in, 156–157
  histoplasmosis in, 193
  osteomyelitis in, 268–269
  perirectal abscess in, 140–141

I

Iliac artery, hemorrhage from, 32–33
Infant
  congenital cystic adenomatoid malformation in, 82–83
  extralobar sequestration in, 60–61
  hepatoblastoma in, 220–221
  teratoma in, 70–71
Infarction, small-bowel, 130–131
Infectious mononucleosis, 320–321
Inferior vena cava, duplication of, 306–307
Inflammatory pseudotumor, of mesentery, 166–167
Inflammatory scar, of lungs, 96–97
Interlobar sequestration, 61

K

Kidneys
  abscess of, 190–191
    postpartum, 198–199
  carcinoma of, 200–201
    deltoid metastasis from, 260–261
  clear-cell carcinoma of, 188–189
  hemorrhage of, 206–207
  mesoblastic nephroma of, 194–195
  mixed follicular-cell lymphoma of, 196–197
  non-Hodgkin lymphoma of, 208–209, 286–287
  perinephric hemorrhage of, 206–207
  postpartum inflammation of, 198–199
  subcapsular hemorrhage of, 206–207
  transplantation of, 14–15
Krukenberg tumor, 180–181

L

Laparoscopic cholecystectomy, complications of, 124–125
Laryngotracheobronchial papillomatosis, 98–99
Laser therapy, for esophageal cancer, 168–169
Leiomyosarcoma, 306–307
Lipoma, 68–69
Liposarcoma, 302–303
Liver
  abscess of, 150–151
  carcinoma of, 242–243
    atrial extension of, 30–31
    multifocal, 238–239, 252–253
    portal-vein invasion by, 218–219
    recurrence of, 226–227, 234–235
  cavernous hemangioma of, 236–237
  focal nodular hyperplasia of, 214–215
  hepatoblastoma of, 220–221
  laceration of, 124–125
  lymphoma of, 216–217
  metastases to, 162–163, 200–201
    from adenocarcinoma, 246–247
    from breast carcinoma, 230–231
    from carcinoid tumor, 244–245
    from colon carcinoma, 228–229, 240–241
    from uterine leiomyosarcoma, 306–307
  nodular regenerative hyperplasia of, 224–225
  normal, 212–213
  pseudolesion of, 250–251, 254–255
  radiation injury to, 232–233
  sarcoidosis of, 316–217
Lumbar artery, hemorrhage from, 26–27
Lungs
  adenocarcinoma of, 74–75, 84–85, 94–95
  anaplastic carcinoma of, 110–111
  embolism of, 100–101
  empyema of, 114–115
  fibrosis of, 76–77
  inflammatory scar of, 96–97
  necrotizing pneumonia of, 118–119
  nodule of, 97
  non-Hodgkin lymphoma of, 106–107

papillomatosis of, 98–99
  radiation injury to, 76–77
  small-cell carcinoma of, 92–93, 102–103
  solitary nodule of, 84–85
  squamous cell carcinoma of, 90–91
Lymph nodes
  in breast cancer, 116–117
  in Castleman's disease, 86–87
  in Hodgkin disease, 64–65
  in melanoma, 72–73
  in small-cell carcinoma, 103
  in thymic carcinoma, 88–89
Lymphangioma, 202–203
Lymphoblastic lymphoma, 66–67
Lymphoma
  follicular-cell, 196–197
  hepatic, 216–217
  lymphoblastic, 66–67
  non-Burkitt's, 142–143
  non-Hodgkin
    of kidneys, 208–209, 286–287
    of pancreas, 286–287
Lysosomal storage disease, 318–319

M

Mediastinal collateral vessels, 56–57
Mediastinum
  Castleman's disease of, 86–87
  hematoma of, 112–113
  mass of, 66–67, 72–73
  non-Hodgkin lymphoma of, 106–107
  post-traumatic, 112–113
Melanoma
  adrenal metastases from, 308–309
  mediastinal, 72–73
Mesentery, inflammatory pseudotumor of, 166–167
Mesoblastic nephroma, 194–195
Metastases
  adrenal, from melanoma, 308–309
  bone, from bladder carcinoma, 266–267
  cardiac, 30–31
  deltoid, from renal-cell tumor, 260–261
  hepatic, 162–163, 200–201
    from adenocarcinoma, 246–247
    from breast carcinoma, 230–231
    from carcinoid tumor, 244–245
    from colon carcinoma, 162–163, 228–229, 240–241
    from uterine leiomyosarcoma, 306–307
  peritoneal, from colon carcinoma, 144–145
  pulmonary, 116–117
Microcystic adenoma, 282–283
Mixed follicular-cell lymphoma, 196–197
Motor vehicle accident
  abdominal hemorrhage with, 146–147
  mediastinal hematoma with, 112–113
  splenic rupture with, 314–315
  sternal fracture with, 112–113
Muscle, metastatic carcinoma of, 260–261
Mycobacterium avium, in esophagitis, 157
Mycobacterium avium complex, in esophagitis, 157

Mycotic aneurysm
    of hepatic artery, 256–257
    of pulmonary artery, 62–63
    of thoracic aorta, 10–11
Myelolipoma, 203
Myxoma, atrial, 4–5

N

Nephroma, mesoblastic, 194–195
Neuroblastoma, 108–109, 186–187
Neuroendocrine tumor, of pancreas,
        300–301
Neurofibromatosis, 176–177
Nodule, pulmonary, 84–85, 97
Non-Burkitt's lymphoma, 142–143
Non-Hodgkin lymphoma, 106–107
    of kidneys, 208–209, 286–287
    of pancreas, 286–287

O

Osteomyelitis
    in acquired immunodeficiency
        syndrome, 268–269
    of sternoclavicular joint, 264–265

P

Pancreas
    carcinoma of
        arterial encasement in, 274–275,
            278–281, 288–293, 296–299
        venous occlusion in, 284–285
    cystadenoma of, 276–277
    liposarcoma compression of, 302–303
    microcystic adenoma of, 282–283
    neuroendocrine tumor of, 300–301
    non-Hodgkin lymphoma of, 286–287
    normal, 272–273
    small ductal adenocarcinoma of, 294–295
Papillomatosis, laryngotracheobronchial,
        98–99
Pleura
    anaplastic carcinoma of, 110–111
    lipoma of, 68–69
    neoplastic invasion of, 74–75
    non-Hodgkin lymphoma of, 106–107
Pleural effusion, 28–29, 80–81, 114–115
Pneumonia, necrotizing, 118–119
Pneumonitis, radiation, 76–77
Portal vein, 2–3
    hepatocellular carcinoma invasion of,
        218–219
Pregnancy, pyelonephritis after, 198–199
Pseudoaneurysm, gluteal, 6–7
Pseudolesion, hepatic, 250–251, 254–255
Pseudomembranous colitis, 148–149

Pseudomonas osteomyelitis, in acquired
        immunodeficiency syndrome,
        268–269
Pseudotumor, inflammatory, of mesentery,
        166–167
Pulmonary artery
    adenocarcinoma invasion of, 94–95
    catheter breakage in, 42–43
    mycotic aneurysm of, 62–63
Pulmonary embolism, 28–29, 100–101
    post-traumatic, 46
Pyelonephritis, postpartum, 198–199

R

Radiation, hepatic injury by, 232–233
Radiation gastritis, 138–139
Radiation pneumonitis, 76–77
Renal artery (arteries)
    in aortic aneurysm, 36–37
    aortic dissection into, 52–53
    normal, 14–15
    occlusion of, 50–51
    reimplantation of, 48–49
    stenosis of, 54–55
    stent of, thrombus in, 8–9
Retroperitoneum, testicular carcinoma
        metastases of, 310–311
Ribs, Hodgkin disease of, 262–263

S

Sarcoidosis, 316–217
Sarcoma, spindle-cell, 78–79
Scar, inflammatory, 96–97
Sigmoid colon
    Crohn's disease of, 150–151
    perforation of, 148–149
Small bowel
    carcinoid tumor of, 244–245
    infarction of, 130–131
    non-Burkitt's lymphoma of, 142–143
    obstruction of, 136–137
        Crohn's disease in, 154–155
Small ductal adenocarcinoma, 294–295
Small-cell carcinoma, pulmonary, 92–93,
        102–103
Spindle-cell sarcoma, 78–79
Spine, Hodgkin disease of, 262–263
Spleen
    Gaucher disease of, 318–319
    normal, 212–213
    rupture of, 314–315
    sarcoidosis of, 316–217
    subcapsular hematoma of, 320–321
Splenic artery, tumor encasement of,
        288–291

Splenic vein, occlusion of, 288–291
Sponge, postsurgical retention of, 104–105
Squamous cell carcinoma, pulmonary,
        90–91
Staphylococcus aureus, empyema with,
        80–81
Staphylococcus endocarditis, pulmonary
        artery aneurysm with, 62–63
Stenosis, of renal artery, 54–55
Stent
    endoluminal
        of abdominal aortic aneurysm, 18–21
        of thoracic aorta rupture, 46–47
        of thoracic aortic aneurysm, 24–25,
            34–35
    renal-artery, thrombus in, 8–9
Sternoclavicular joint, osteomyelitis of,
        264–265
Sternum, fracture of, 112–113
Stricture, esophageal, 135
Superior vena cava syndrome, 56–57
Surgical sponge, postsurgical retention of,
        104–105

T

Teratoma, in infant, 70–71
Testis, carcinoma of, retroperitoneal
        recurrence of, 310–311
Thoracic aorta
    aneurysm of, 34–35, 44–45
        endoluminal stent graft of, 24–25
    dissection of, 28–29, 52–53
    mycotic aneurysm of, 10–11
Thrombus
    of heart, 16–17
    in renal-artery stent, 8–9
Thymus carcinoma, 88–89
Trauma
    abdominal hemorrhage with, 146–147
    aortic rupture with, 46–47
    mediastinal hematoma with, 112–113
    splenic rupture with, 314–315
    sternal fracture with, 112–113

U

Ulcer
    of abdominal aorta, 22–23
    gastric
        Helicobacter pylori in, 165
        perforation of, 132–133
Ureter, calculus of, 172–173, 182–183
Uterus, leiomyosarcoma of, 306–307

V

Von Recklinghausen disease, 176–177

ISBN 0-395-16681-0

9 780395 166819